New Angles on
Dementia
What everyone needs to know

By Torben Riise

with

Esther Davidsen &

Maria Tønnersen

New Angles on Dementia

What everyone needs to know

By Torben Riise, PhD, MBA

with
Esther Davidsen, MA, MBA, EMCC
Maria Tønnersen, RN, BA

New Angles on Dementia is written and edited by Torben Riise with contributions from Esther Davidsen and Maria Tønnersen, and four other writers.

All rights reserved. © 2020 Torben Riise
Phoenix/Arizona - USA
ISBN:9798515336134

Dedication

This book is an edited collection of articles first published online in Denmark during 2019-20. These articles are based on the latest research into many aspects of dementia and are written to be easily accessible to lay people as well as private and public caregivers at all levels.

The book is dedicated to everyone with an interest in dementia, whether they already have the disease or want to know about it and be prepared for a life with dementia if they would get it at some point in time.

By sharing knowledge, insight, and advice about dementia, it is the hope of the writers that the book inspires and empowers the readers to improve the quality of their life if the disease strikes a member of the family.

Acknowledgement

This book might not have reached its completion, and certainly not its final form, had it not been for the assistance and encouragement of several individuals.

First of all, I want to thank my partners in Denmark, Esther Davidsen and Maria Tønnersen for their support in getting this book together. It is based on a Danish version of the book, which was published in June 2021 in Denmark. Esther and Maria comprise the core group behind an online information universe dedicated to inform, educate, inspire, and serve people with an interest in the field of dementia.

Further, I want to thank several avid readers for input and comments, in particular Pamela Lajoie and Ann Doucette for their exceptional review and many constructive comments that greatly contributed to giving the book the presentation it has today.

In the background, the technical input provided by Brant Herbert on the use of a sophisticated writing application greatly facilitated the writing and editing process in a way I could never had achieved on my own. Thanks . . . again!

These contributions have improved the readability of this book. Any shortcomings are entirely a result of my own limitations and do not reflect upon the contributions of these individuals.

I thank you all!

CONTENTS

INTRODUCTION   side 9

SECTION 1: WORTH THINKING ABOUT . . . includes some general but nonetheless very important considerations about dementia and people with dementia:

1. Demented or person with dementia   page 14
   - language difference with great significance
2. Dementia and consciousness   page 23
3. Dementia and Alzheimer's
   - What are the differences?   page 26

SECTION 2: LIVING WITH DEMENTIA . . . includes articles on everyday topics and problems that the vast majority will face in the course of the development of the dementia disease:

1. Dementia friendly housing   page 32
2. COVID-19   page 34
3. Next of kin   page 36
4. Good conversations   page 40
5. Independence   page 43

SECTION 3: LIFESTYLE ISSUES . . . covers lifestyle issues, i.e. areas where we have great control over our physical, mental, and cognitive health:

1. Risk of dementia   page 48
2. Diets   page 50

3. The Mediterranean Diet — page 54
4. Olive oil — page 57
5. Exercise and dementia — page 60
6. Exercise as a lifestyle — page 63
7. Exercise - 5 good pieces of advice — page 66
8. Exercise - get started — page 68
9. Exercise without exercising — page 71
10. Overweight — page 74
11. Weight loss — page 76
12. Sleep — page 78
13. Dehydration — page 82

SECTION 4: WORTH KNOWING - SPECIAL SUBJECTS . . . includes articles on what happens to a person who has dementia at various levels:

1. Blood test/Alzheimer's — page 86
2. Blood pressure — page 88
3. Pollution — page 92
4. Better memory — page 94
5. Immune system — page 97
6. Inflammations — page 101
7. L-serine — page 103
8. Medical drugs - be careful! — page 105
9. New medicine for Alzheimer's — page 107
10. Medicine for dementia - do they work? — page 109
11. Menopause — page 111
12. Dizziness — page 114
13. Tests or not — page 116
14. Vaccination — page 119

SECTION 5: ABOUT THE BRAIN AND OUR SENSES . . . includes articles on the brain and our senses; the articles are primarily aimed at those who are curious to know "what actually is happening in the body and in the brain" when the disease develops:

1. Dementia and consciousness	page 122
2. Lewy's Body dementia	page 123
3. Myths about the brain	page 127
4. Senses and body functions	page 130
5. Hearing	page 133
6. Vision and hearing	page 136

SECTION 6: SEX AND INTIMACY . . . includes articles on sex and intimacy and the changes, challenges, and opportunities that arise when dementia becomes part of cohabitation:

1. Introduction	page 140
2. Sex - Del I: Changes	page 144
3. Sex - Del II: Challenges	page 148
4. Sex - Del III: Possibilities	page 153
5. Sex or no sex	page 158

SECTION 7: ABOUT THE AUTHORS . . . gives a brief introduction to the authors.

1. About the authors	page 164
2. Contact information	page 165

INTRODUCTION
Knowledge is power!

If we want to take control of our lives and the challenges we face, it requires that we have the necessary knowledge to do so. This is especially true in a field such as dementia.

Dementia is a group of incurable diseases that can severely affect and debilitate both the individual and his/her family - and society.

Dementia is one of the biggest causes of disability and loss of independence among elderly people, and it is the third leading cause of death in wealthy countries (1 in 3 seniors over 65).

The disease develops slowly - starting as early as the late 40s/early 50s - and manifests itself much later in life. In other words, it can be underway long before we know it, and when we get the diagnosis, there is "no way back".

Against this background, everything one can do to delay the onset or possibly completely prevent the disease is invaluable.

This is where **knowledge** comes in.

This book is about knowledge of what the disease is, knowledge about what individuals, their families, and caretakers can do to get the best out of the situation, and, above all, knowledge about what a person who does *not* have the disease can do to improve the chances of avoiding it in the future!

With this in mind, the book is dedicated to the many people who want easy access to knowledge about a wide range of topics on dementia.

Let's take a closer look at these large groups.

First, there are more than 6.2 million people in the U.S. with age-related dementia. It is estimated (health care officials in the U.S. and Europe) that for every person with dementia, there are 4-5 family members directly impacted by the disease. That is another

25-30 million people. As the population and lifespan increase, these numbers are expected to double by 2040.

Secondly, there are more than 115 million people in the U.S. over the age of 50, of which

- 62 million are between 50 and 64; among them, 1 in 6 women and 1 in 10 men will get dementia, and
- 53 million are over 65; among them, 1 in 5 women and 1 in 8 men will get dementia

Together, that means that in the next 15-20 years, more than 17 million people will be diagnosed with the disease. The cost to society of caring for this many people is estimated to exceed $350 Bn, not including the value of the time of *free* caregivers (estimated to be $250 Bn) - all in 2020 value.

And finally, there's a group of professionals in the private and public sector who in various ways are involved in the care of people with dementia.

So, in total there are 120-140 million people who will benefit from the information in this book, *either* because they have the disease or know they are at risk of developing the disease, *or* simply because they might want to be well informed about it in case they should be diagnosed with it in the future.

As mentioned, there is no cure for this disease yet, so a key aspect of the articles included in the book is to highlight *what one can do* to delay (i.e. reduce the risk of) the onset of the disease and live a good life with it, should they get it.

We have strived to bring articles that are both down-to-earth and practical as well as have a high professional and scientific content, without being difficult to understand. The backgrounds of the authors (see p. 164) are in dementia care, nursing, biotechnology, and healthcare administration - but none of them are medical doctors.

Therefore, we want to emphasize that these articles do not replace consultations with your own doctor or the professional staff in municipalities.

At the same time, we want to emphasize that because we are all different, none of the solutions or advice presented on these pages will apply to everyone.

Use the book as an empowerment of your life and as an inspiration for whatever you may want to discuss with your doctor/professional.

The articles are grouped into the 6 main sections indexed above. Each of them can be read independently.

We hope you find this book useful. You can always contact the authors with questions, comments, or topics you would like to be addressed in future updates (see contact page in SECTION 7, p. 165).

June 2021
The authors/editors

SECTION 1: WORTH THINKING ABOUT

CONTENTS

1. Demented or person with dementia   page 14
   - language difference with great significance

2. Dementia and consciousness   page 23

3. Dementia and Alzheimer's
   - What are the differences?   page 26

'Demented' or 'person with dementia'
- a language difference of great significance

Do you say "demented" or "person with dementia?"
Does it matter at all whether we say one thing or the other? We know what we're talking about. But below we explain why it makes a big difference.

Because what we are saying always makes a big difference, we hope you will read this article with great attention and consider the recommendations given at the end.

This topic has two perspectives:
- The individual perspective that emanates from the people who have a dementia illness close to home (the sick and their relatives, friends, workplace and the like)
- The perspective of society *and* the professionals in the field of dementia.

###

THE INDIVIDUAL PERSPECTIVE

Things are evolving—thankfully.
In the field of dementia, we have seen a development over time, which has gone from focusing on the *disease* to focusing on *the person* who has it and on 'what it's like to have the disease.'

This shift in perspective and the derived effects are still underway and it will take quite some time before we reach the goal. Below, we have summarized these aspects (according to the British psychologist and professor, Tom Kitwood):

The old perspective
We say 'demented people' - We focus on and treat dementia - We consider inappropriate behavior as a sign of illness and then treat it - We focus on pathology and treatment - We distinguish between professional and private relationships - We focus on reality orientation - The professionals are the experts and their efforts are based on the knowledge learned.

The new perspective
We say 'people with dementia' - We focus on the whole person and on the whole body's functioning - We consider inappropriate behavior as a sign of communication and adapt our efforts accordingly - We focus on life history, habits, and values on an equal footing with pathology - We use ourselves as tools for sincere relationships - We meet people with dementia in their world and recognize their experiences - It is the people with dementia and their relatives who are experts and who show the way for the professionals.

Why this shift?
As mentioned, the old concept of 'dement' is a result of a *disease perspective* that we are trying to move away from. The phrase '*people* with dementia' helps us remember what we are heading towards.

Back to the question. Why do we even discuss how we use words and concepts?

We all view the world based on our experiences. We carry mental baggage with us, which characterizes the way we are. In relation to Kitwood's list above, our baggage is primarily filled up with the old perspective. It is natural and predictable. That perspective is based on the traditions that have prevailed within the treatment area, within the media, and in society.

In many ways we can say we have worked around the individual. We have focused on investigation, diagnosis, and treatment of the disease, incl. vaccines, in recent years. That has taken us a long way in terms of how well we treat the disease. But we forgot the individual along the way.

For example . . .

Are "dementia cities" a good idea?

We have established dementia cities, which in many ways make good sense, solve a major security aspect, and satisfy a certain social need. But, the devil's advocate would say dementia cities are precisely a result of a stigmatization of people with dementia. We pack them away so that we ourselves are not disturbed or bothered, so that we do not have to deal with them and think about them. Out of sight, out of mind!

In other words, we reflect our society is not designed to accommodate people with dementia, and that our attitude is that they are unwanted. And here comes the most important thing:

The result of this is that people with dementia face this attitude of working around them, of making decisions on their behalf, of taking their self-esteem away from them!

Ouch! Shame on us!

It takes a lot of effort to reverse this view. The attitudes in society are not that easy to change. But we're making progress.

Fortunately, we find that the change of perspective creates value immediately. Just like any other human being, people with dementia need to feel respected; they need to feel that we who do *not* have the disease, need them; they need to feel that we respect *their* way of experiencing the world; and that we need the things *they* can teach us.

A *sincere* attitude

If we return to "the new perspective" list above, the central focus is the point that "We use ourselves to create sincere relationships" with people with dementia. It places great demands on both relatives and professionals.

It requires that we sincerely are curious about each other, that we sincerely are working on getting better at creating relationships.

The word *sincerely* points to the need to face *our own* prejudices and deal with them if we are to create the new perspective.

This was clearly expressed in a recent study (Jacob Birkler - former chairman of the Danish Ethics Council - Survey 2020), in which he concludes that "it is not the lack of memory that was the worst part of having dementia . . . it is *the way* the outside world reacts to the lack of memory."

Ouch again!

At the same time, the adjustment process will teach us an incredible amount about ourselves and about our way of being, about our own relationships with people with dementia.

It is an incredibly apt example of the difference between the two perspectives we mentioned in the introduction, that the outside world focuses on the disease and not on the human being.

What can we do?

We all want to be wanted and need to be needed . . . as a life partner, a family member, a friend, as an employee, or a volunteer. We have roles in many contexts, which help create our identity and values in life.

People who suffer from dementia experience that these roles change markedly after they get the disease. It is a natural consequence of getting an illness that affects you as profoundly as a dementia does.

Many have to stop working, many experience that their friends drop out, leisure and social activities also become difficult to maintain. And we tend to explain it all from the point of view of dementia. But wouldn't it be exciting to turn it all upside down - change the perspective to assume that it is the person with dementia who has the right to define *their* reality? As a result, the rest of us could try to adapt to a greater degree.

For example:

What if the workplace would . . .
- create space for an employee with dementia, adapt tasks, frameworks, meeting times, etc. to fit the employee's reality?
- insist that the employee with dementia has a value no matter what framework the employee needs?
- keep in touch with the employee throughout the course of the illness
- educate colleagues to see the value in the person with dementia?

How would that be experienced?

What about our own situation?

The same change of perspective is important in close relationships with a cohabitant/relative, but that, too, is difficult. It takes energy and effort to be a part of the necessary development and change ourself along the way with a person who develops dementia.

Acquiring this disease is associated with sadness, powerlessness and loneliness. Changing the perspective requires we embrace the changes in our partner and "go into combat training" to see the person behind the disease, see the resources that are always present in them.

So, similar to the workplace questions above, think about:

What if . . .
- relatives find new qualities in relation to the person with dementia?
- dementia provides an opportunity for more peace and presence in the relationship?
- dementia gives new perspectives on how life can be lived?
- dementia teaches us to be far better at living in the moment?

How would that situation be experienced?

The situation of the caregiving relative

We know how our own mood and energy rub off on other people. As a party in a relationship, you naturally become impacted by *other* people's attitudes and perceptions about what it is like to have dementia, and you take these attitudes and perceptions with you into the close relationship and now view the person *in the light of the surroundings*. It is very important to be on guard against this impact because it makes it particularly difficult to change your perspective.

You have to cope with the grief *and* live with the challenges and frustrations. To make progress, you must face your own "prejudices" about dementia - and deal with them. You must see the person with dementia as a human being *you* need, see them as someone who has the resources and right to be in the world *the way they now are*, a person with a disease and whatever comes with it.

If we as relatives can find meaning in the process, can take care of ourselves, can make sure we "refuel" when needed, then we can actually influence the dementia process positively.

It is easier said than done, and therefore it is a journey one cannot make alone.

You have to get help and support, and you will have to swallow your pride along the way. It's difficult for most people to meet others on *their* terms and at the same time help them in the transition. But it is those of us *who are not affected* by dementia who have the resources to meet people with dementia in their world - if we dare. But the rewards are great.

The rewards

For the person with dementia, these changes in perspective will make a big difference.

It will give them an experience of acceptance and existential justification. We all have felt like an outsider, felt misunderstood, and without purpose in life. But it eases when we orient ourselves towards new goals, create new relationships, and redefine our values.

We can achieve this by changing our perspective.

Advice

We encourage anyone who is in contact with a person with dementia to discuss all these perspectives with them. It's the only way you can be sure that *you* know how the person with dementia experiences his situation, which is different in each case. And it is the only way you will know what and how you can contribute to make the situation easier and increase the quality of life for all concerned.

It is no small task, but it is worth the effort.

Additional material: We encourage you to read the article *Dementia and consciousness* (p. 23, below) with the theme 'is anyone home?' It provides a thought-provoking insight into the consciousness of a person with dementia, which relatives and carers must not overlook.

###

SOCIETY'S PERSPECTIVE

In addition to the human aspects of this shift in perspective, there is a societal perspective of similar importance.

General problems

Think about this issue:

Has anyone ever asked a pupil/student what he or she thinks about the teaching, the class and study schedule, the content, the relevance, etc.? Has anyone ever asked an immigrant about his or her views on integration, on the desire to become a citizen in his/her new country, or about what he or she needs most to fit in? Has anyone ever asked an inmate about his or her views on rehabilitation, on life as an inmate, on what he or she needs to re-socialize?

The answers are no, or at best, rarely!

We almost always ignore to involve the people who are directly affected by the systems we establish around them, and in the process cut ourselves off from valuable information that these people can provide to other citizens and communities.

In other words, we have turned them into "objects," into data points in the "statistics" we rely on when we organize resources, make new programs, and so on.

We therefore have no idea if these programs work *for the individual*.

The dementia attitudes

As explained below, the same is true of people with dementia.

Society has many different parameters to navigate and measure itself against. It is often said that a society is characterized by the way it treats its weakest citizens.

For the past many years, we have worked to create better conditions for some of the weakest in our society, including people with dementia. We have qualified the staff, enlightened the community, made dementia friends, held dementia weeks, created dementia villages, and much more—all with the best intention of improving the lives of people affected by dementia.

But what if it doesn't work for the person with dementia or if some of the initiatives have the opposite effect?

Negative social psychology

Tom Kitwood has written about what he calls 'negative social psychology.' This concept covers, among other things, the stigma, disapproval and objectification many people with dementia experience, who in turn cease to represent a societal value, and, so to speak, are "judged out". Our social structures support this. We make systems that work *around* the person with dementia, that measure the framework around them (documentation, dementia-friendly design, consumption of medication, number of uses of force, etc.). We do not see them, we do not experience what happens to them when they get the disease, do not really focus on how it is experienced *to have dementia* and how to thrive with it.

A practical initiative

In England, they have opened "The Restaurant That Makes Mistakes," a place that exemplifies how recognition, employment and inclusion in communities can be used to dismantle negative, social psychology about people with dementia and give them a sense of being valuable to the society.

When mistakes and neglect occur, we always talk about the lack of resources—and that may, of course, often be the case, but not always. It is very much a question of human vision, about how we recognize people with dementia, talk to them, be together with them, and support them in having a meaningful life.

It requires much more than just saying "I meet them at eye level." It requires that we regard people with dementia *as equal*, as people with the same social justification and needs as we ourselves have.

It is an encouraging development that will surely continue.

Sources: "The Restaurant That Makes Mistakes"
see https://www.alzheimers.org.uk/restaurant-that-makes-mistakes.

Dementia and consciousness

Below, we look at dementia and consciousness and answer the question: "Is anyone home" - implying "behind the empty shell."

When we are in the unfortunate situation that a family member has advanced dementia, it is important to be aware of the fact that a person with dementia actually has the same consciousness as before the disease struck.

What is consciousness?

Consciousness has been the subject of countless philosophical considerations for two thousand years. And consciousness has been the subject of intense research since Sigmund Freud around 1900 gave psychoanalysis/psychology a place next to major research areas such as physics, chemistry and biology.

Excellent researchers in many fields go wrong, in the opinion of the writer, when they try to define and uncover *what* consciousness is and, even more so, *where it can be found*.

Very briefly, even if they don't quite know what consciousness is, these scientists are sure that they one day (soon?) will find it "somewhere in the brain." That's the worrying part because consciousness is not something one can find.

We will take a closer look at that.

What consciousness is not

Let us first establish that "consciousness" is not a physical phenomenon! Therefore, one cannot "find" consciousness - in the brain or anywhere else in the same way we can find physical objects!

When we see brain waves on an MRI scan, we often think they are pictures of our thoughts or of our "consciousness." In reality, what we see is a picture of *where and how the brain works* in a given situation, i.e. which brain cells and electrical impulses are involved in implementing a given activity (incl. thinking).

This leads to the important conclusion that *one doesn't lose consciousness when one "loses consciousness"* by, for example, hitting one's head against something hard.

If that *were* the case, it would require two follow-up questions,

(1) Where does the consciousness go when we 'lose it'—and

(2) how does it come back when we 'regain' it?

But since that's not the case, the question becomes, "What is it then, that we lose?"

The brain and the consciousness - two different things

The answer is actually quite simple. *You lose the brain's ability to work!*

Our thoughts (our so-called inner dialogue) are a result (output) of the brain's processing of the content of the consciousness (input). The brain works in the same way as a slide projector, which converts a digital input (equivalent to consciousness input) into a visual output (the image on the screen, equivalent to our thoughts that we might express).

Neither more nor less.

What does this have to do with dementia?

There are many profound and fascinating aspects of this concept of consciousness. One of them—and in this context, the most important—is that it is the *brain's ability* to process input from consciousness, which is gradually lost when a person gets dementia/Alzheimer's. It is not a loss of consciousness!

A similar aspect is that when "we forget something," it is the brain's *access* to the memory content in the consciousness that is impaired, *not* that the memory content (consciousness) is not there anymore. In other words, it is the physical changes in the brain that gradually reduce the brain's ability to *process* the content (e.g. remembering or performing other cognitive functions).

Why is that so important?
When we understand this, the answer to the question, "is anyone home" when we talk about a person with advanced dementia/Alzheimer's, is "Yes! There *is* someone home." A person with advanced dementia/Alzheimer's has the same consciousness as he/she had before getting dementia!

Knowing this makes it no less tragic to see a human being slip away from you. Quite the contrary.

But it gives people in the patient's environment a special obligation to rethink the problem of whether it pays to visit mor father/mother, because "he/she can't remember I've just been there —or even remember who I am."

Visiting people with dementia is often one of the things family and friends dread the most.

But we must remember that even though the brain cannot express what the consciousness wants to express, many people with dementia experience great value of a visit, feel they are not forgotten, that they are not hidden away. We all develop positive, biological reactions (in the amygdala of the brain and on the cellular and hormonal levels) when we are together with people we care about.

It is no different for a person with dementia.

The importance of this was established in the study mentioned above (*Demented or a person with dementia*, p.14), which showed that for people with dementia, the (negative) reactions of the environment are perceived as much harder to deal with than the very fact that they forget things.

Dignity in the treatment
This aspect of the dementia disease can be difficult to get acquainted with. But it teaches us that people with dementia should be treated with dignity and given a sense of caring for them, that they are not alone, and so on.

It is undeniably a very big and difficult task - but it is worth completing.

Dementia and Alzheimer's

The words Dementia and Alzheimer's are often used as if they are one and the same disease. However, dementia covers a number of cognitive diseases, of which Alzheimer's is the most common. Although there are some overlap between these diseases, they all have their individual characteristics.

Below, we cover the four types of dementia that comprise 95-98% of the cases and look at the differences.

General facts

- Dementia is a common term for several diseases that affect the cognitive functions, such as memory, attention, communication, recognition of otherwise familiar objects, reasoning, sense of time, etc. Emotional life can also be affected by a dementia disease.

- People used to describe the reduced ability to think, concentrate, or remember as "*senility.*" Being senile is an old-fashioned terminology. The medical profession increasingly use the term 'minor or major "neurocognitive disorder due to [e.g.] Alzheimer's disease." For the sake of simplicity, in this book we use 'dementia' and 'Alzheimer's' whenever we refer to cognitive diseases in general.

- Everyone can be affected by a dementia disease, but the vast majority of the people diagnosed with dementia are people over 60-65 years.

- Although dementia is predominantly found in older people, *age is not the cause* of dementia! Admittedly, with age comes a certain forgetfulness, a certain impairment of physiological functions, and a certain deterioration of our senses. It is normal and *not* in themselves signs of dementia.

- Although we often find people with dementia in the same families, there is not (yet) any proven sign of heredity.

The four most common forms of dementia are:
- Alzheimer's accounts for approx. 60-70% of all cases; it is characterized by an accumulation of plaque between the brain cells *and* entanglement of protein inside the brain cells; women are tree times more likely to get Alzheimer's than men are (about three out of four cases)
- Lewy's Body Dementia, makes up approx. 10-20% of all cases and often occurs together with Parkinson's; Lewy's is characterized by an accumulation of proteins inside the brain cells, which prevents the normal communication between the cells; men are far more likely to get Lewy's than women are.
- Vascular dementia, which accounts for approx. 10-15% of all cases, differ from other dementia diseases because it does not occur in or between the brain cells, but is a result of problems with the blood supply to the brain (often caused by atherosclerosis, blood clots, and bleeding in the brain).
- Fronto-temporal dementia amounts to approx. 5% of all cases; it attacks the frontal lobes of the brain; therefore, FTD often leads to personality changes, which can be a strain on the family and at work. There are often also problems with speaking and understanding speech.

There are, as mentioned, overlaps between these diseases and the factors that lead to them. The actual mechanisms by which they develop are not well known but are being intensely researched. There is not yet a cure for dementia, although certain types of medication can alleviate the symptoms and make the development 'milder.' You can read more about the latter in the article *Medicine and dementia - do they work* in Section 4 below.

Symptoms of dementia

Below we list the symptoms of dementia (in particular Alzheimer's).

The most common ones are that the person increasingly forgets things like appointments, names of people they have known all their life. Later, it may be forgetfulness about eating or taking one's medication. Other symptoms are confusion about time and place, difficulty making good decisions, changes in one's personality and emotional life, as well as difficulty coping with practical tasks that have been accomplished many times before.

The progression of the disease is typically described in seven stages:

Stage 1: Very few symptoms, incipient forgetfulness
Stage 2: Minor memory loss, forgetfulness with names, impaired concentration
Stage 3: Forgetfulness regarding new information, decrease in work performance, difficulty in planning future activities, problems with organization, repetition of questions
Stage 4: Difficulty with complex activities, unable to plan time and activities, depression, withdrawal, avoiding challenging situations
Stage 5: Difficulty remembering home address and telephone number, need for assistance with cooking, disorientation regarding time and place, declining personal hygiene
Stage 6: Need for assistance with dressing, forgetfulness with names of close family members, changes in personality incl. hallucinations and paranoia, incipient need for constant monitoring, and help with all personal hygiene
Stage 7: Inability to speak or answer sensibly, failing muscle control, difficulty sitting up, beginning difficulty swallowing food and drink.

Be aware of changes

It is important to remember that if you experience some of the symptoms above, it is not a given you are in the initial stage of dementia. Failing memory can also be a natural consequence of getting older. Mind you, 1as we age, all people lose brain capacity in a slow and imperceptible process. Most people have ways to compensate for that without the major dementia symptoms, precisely because the process is sufficiently slow. It can also be a sign of other conditions, such as stress, depression, or other medical issues. It can even be the result of a really long day.

However, *combined,* it may be a sign of dementia.

Therefore, it is important to keep an eye on the symptoms. If you—or someone close to you—notice that something is not quite as it used to be, that you forget things or experience other symptoms *more often* than usual, then you should contact your doctor.

Sources:
Karger International (www.karger.com/Article/Pdf/333812)
Alzheimer International (https://tinyurl.com/y4t5g4vf)
WHO (https://tinyurl.com/y4t5g4vf)
Relating to plaque/beta-amyloid: https://tinyurl.com/y4xvehkz
https://www.who.int/news-room/fact-sheets/detail/dementia
https://www.dementiasociety.org

SECTION 2: LIVING WITH DEMENTIA

CONTENTS

1. Dementia friendly housing   page 32
2. COVID-19   page 34
3. Next of kin   page 36
4. Good conversations   page 40
5. Independence   page 43

Dementia friendly housing

For a person with dementia, the arrangement of your living space can be a source of great frustration. If you want to avoid stress in everyday life, you can try to rearrange the furniture and other things in your environment.

Avoid frustrations and stress

Too many choices in everyday life make people with dementia frustrated and create unnecessary stress. Once you have adapted your home to a life with dementia, it can give you more energy and lift your spirit because you remove many obstacles.

If you want to understand how a person with dementia experiences stress, you can imagine one of those days when you have no control over anything. A day when the keys are lost when you're about to go for a walk, and you cannot remember where your cell phone is, even though you carry it in your hand, and you on top of it cannot remember how to use it. And then imagine if you cannot remember why you're on your way out the door.

Of course, there are many more aspects of dementia than those described here, but it may give you an idea of some of the challenges a person with dementia faces in the early stages of the disease.

People with dementia face such situations all the time, and they are far more affected by them than the rest of us. Therefore, it is important to create conditions for people with dementia that prevent the stress and frustration of making choices. One of the ways to avoid stress and frustration is by living "dementia-friendly."

Below are 5 simple things you can do to improve your living conditions.

5 simple tips for making your home dementia-friendly
1. Make sure there is adequate lighting throughout the home. Bathrooms in particular are often quite dark
2. Pay attention to level differences on the floor, such as door steps or area rugs
3. Use labels to show what's in the cupboards and drawers
4. Make life as simple as possible, narrow down choices in everyday life.
5. Organize belongings so that they are not filled with things that are not necessary.

COVID-19

We will probably be living with COVID-19 (and its mutations) in society for a long time to come, so we need good advice on COVID-19 in relation to dementia. You may find that some of this has been said before, but it cannot be repeated too often.

1. Most survive COVID-19

We know that people over the age of 60 have a five times higher risk of developing COVID-19 (hereinafter called "covid") as people under the age of 60, and that people over the age of 75/80 have a 10 times higher risk.

Nevertheless, it is important to remember that by far the largest proportion of the elderly — more than 85% —don't have serious complications and 98% survive the disease.

Taking care of a person with Alzheimer's is in itself a big and difficult task, but it is further complicated if the person gets covid.

Due to the risk of infection, contacts with other people should therefore be limited completely or in part. But if the human condition worsens, then how do you handle a doctor's visit?

2. Call the doctor instead of showing up

If you think you or a member of your family has covid, it's recommended not to show up physically in the doctor's office, but call first. Most doctors now have consultations over the Internet or by phone.

In many cases, a caregiver comes home to a person with Alzheimer's. If it is not possible/practical to provide care outdoors, it is important that the caregiver

- checks his/her own temperature before going inside; if it is above 101.5 °F (38.5 °C) the caregiver should not come into contact with a person with Alzheimer's

- washes hands thoroughly
- uses face masks

Face masks are, unfortunately, somewhat of a barrier to communication between people, but this is of particular concern between people with Alzheimer's and their caregivers because the patients cannot see the caregivers' facial expressions, thereby missing out on important visual and emotional cues.

But the use of face masks is nonetheless important. The reason is that dementia weakens the body's immune system (see the article on the Immune System in Section 4, p. 97), so there is an extra reason to be careful.

It is also important that people with dementia learn to avoid touching their face. Maintaining a calm environment and daily routines is also important, especially as society opens up more and more.

3. Eat well, exercise, and get proper sleep

For the sake of good order, it should be mentioned that people with dementia can do a lot to delay the development and reduce the effect of the disease.

Some of the most important factors are a healthy diet (Mediterranean diet plan, p. 54), exercise, and plenty of sleep. We refer to special articles on these factors in Section 4 (p. 85).

PS: Needless to say, other infectious diseases can be challenging, too, so a person with Alzheimer's should adopt the above suggestions in such situations.

Sources:
Information from the Alzheimer's Foundation of America - https://alzfdn.org
https://alz-journals.onlinelibrary.wiley.com/doi/10.1002/alz.12255

Next of kin

"Henry, I already told you twice we're going to the gym this afternoon!"

Do you know the feeling of having to answer the same question over and over again?

Every day.

Or doing your absolute best not to sound annoyed while patiently explaining how the remote control or microwave works - again?

If one of your loved ones has dementia, you probably recognize situations like the above mentioned.

You try to be open about the problems that may be associated with dementia, but it can be frustrating for all parties when the disease takes over. Therefore, we have gathered some advice on how you as a relative of a person with dementia best can handle everyday life issues.

Everyday life with dementia

The person with dementia has difficulty remembering mundane things, and it can be difficult to understand the person because words disappear or are swapped with words of completely different meanings.

In addition, a person with dementia often experiences sensory disturbances that can affect the quality of life in a very negative way (read more about our senses in the three articles in Section 5, p. 121).

Families who deal with dementia have probably already adapted to the new situation and found their own solutions. They make small but important changes and arrangements that make living easier by removing the focus from the negative impacts of the disease.

Get inspired by others

Although self-made solutions often are a good place to start, knowing how others deal with the disease and the challenges it poses can be a great help. It's important to keep in mind that many other families deal with dementia at various degrees, so there's a lot of good advice to take from people who have the experience of a life with the disease. See the article above about dementia-friendly homes (p. 32).

Aids for everyday life

As a relative, you have a desire to help and support the person with dementia manage themselves in the best possible way, so that he or she can maintain a sense of independence. Fortunately, there is a plethora of things that can help structuring life, remembering appointments, helping a person find their way around - *and* being found (using GPS) if they lose their way and cannot find home.

You can ask professionals for advice, but they don't always have up-to-date knowledge because the market constantly evolves.

Use the power of habit

To find simple solutions that can help the person with dementia in his/her life, it is important to remember to start with whatever works for you. Take a look at what habits and routines already exist. Stick to the type of calendar you always have used; make a reusable shopping list with the products and foods you use the most; make sure to put more light up in the home, as dark surroundings make it harder to find things and to find your way around.

Some people put stickers on the on/off button of the remote control or coffee machine, or paint the mailbox in a special color so it's easier to recognize. Others put home-made labels or pictures on cupboards, so you can see/read what's in them, or place their medicine next to the coffee machine so they are reminded to take it.

Research in dementia

As mentioned several times in this book, there is no cure for dementia. Many researchers are currently investigating the origin of dementia in order to find a medical treatment. Until then, people with dementia and their relatives must resort to aids and other solutions that can alleviate their challenges. In the following you will find a wide range of both high- and low-tech aids that can improve your quality of life.

Technology can help

In the high-tech area, you can find apps for smartphones. Through text and pictures, you can easily get an overview of daily chores and appointments, so you and your family can structure your life together.

Besides apps, there are many other high-tech aids on the market.

For example:
- GPS trackers
- Key finder
- Automatic lighting
- Phones with fewer and larger buttons

There are also many low-tech products available. A few examples of low-tech solutions are:
- Colored toilet bowls
- Glass doors in the kitchen cabinets
- Calendars with spiral spine

In both areas, the market is large and there is an aid for almost every need. Your imagination is the only limit.

The vast majority of aids have been developed with the aim of benefiting a wider population group and not just people with dementia.

As relatives of people with dementia, it is a good idea to search the Internet for useful products and services, or to contact local activity centers for people with dementia, or get advice from the dementia consultant in your municipality.

Source: To read more about current research into a cure for dementia, visit https://tinyurl.com/y4lewpy7

Good conversations

Relatives of people with dementia often experience difficulties in communicating with the person as they gradually become a shadow of themselves. Below, we look at what a good conversation is and how you can best establish it.

Below, we list some of the most important ways of communicating in order to have a meaningful and dignified contact with the affected person. There will be days when it's easy and days when it seems impossible. The key is to remember that dementia is not the end of a life of hope, dignity, and initiative.

But one must not ignore the fact that dementia gets worse over time. The person will gradually have more difficulties understanding others and expressing themselves. Therefore, it is good if you as early as possible establish a conversational "format" that the person becomes familiar with.

Clear and 'present' communication

A good conversation is based on 10 important factors:

- **Avoid distractions.** Find a place and time where you can talk together without being disturbed. It allows the mental energy to be focused on the conversation.
- **Speak clearly and naturally with a warm and calm voice.** Avoid "baby talk" or other "condescending" ways of expressing yourself.
- **Always refer to people using their names.** Avoid using "he/she," "him/her," and "they/them," when the conversation is about others. That is confusing. Instead, use their names. Names are also important when you greet each other, e.g. "Hi Grandma, it's me, John," is far better than "Hi Grandma, it's me."

- **Talk about only one thing at a time**. People with dementia are often unable to talk about several things at one time. They get mixed up and confused.

Body language and physical contact is good
- **Use non-verbal cues.** Eye contact and smiles help to "warm up" and make the conversation easier and more relaxed. The same goes for physical contact, such as holding hands. Listening to music together has a similar effect. These methods are also a good preparation for a possible future situation when this is the only way you can communicate.
- **Copy the body language of the person with dementia.** One can build bridges and trust by copying the non-verbal gestures the person uses. If he/she raises eyebrows, smiles, puffs his cheeks, pats his hands, etc., do the same.
- **Listen actively**. If any of what the person with dementia is saying does not make sense, say it to them in a kind and positive way. Also be aware that such a person often has fluid boundaries when they talk or make comments. They often mix stories and time periods together in a single sequence. Instead of paying so much attention to the present or the past and rather accept the process *as it is told*, self-confidence and communication are strengthened.
- **Avoid wordplay**. The conversation will not progress very far or last very long if we correct any incorrect statement. It is OK to let certain mistakes and misunderstandings pass.
- **Have patience**. Give the person with dementia extra time to process what you say and plenty of time to answer the questions you ask. Avoid getting frustrated.
- **Realize there are good days and bad days.** Although the general trend in the development of dementia is a gradual deterioration, a person with dementia - like everyone else - has good days and bad days.

Do not give up.

When conversations become more difficult, do not close the door for the positive experiences that being with family and friends - with or without conversation - represents for the person with dementia.

Read the article in Section 1 about *Dementia and consciousness*, p. 23) There is a lot of inspiration in that article that applies to the points mentioned here.

Share your experiences of conversations with people with dementia

If you have experiences - good or not so good - that you think might help others in their communication with a family member who has dementia, send us a few words about it.

Get more ideas in the article on *Next of kin* above, and don't forget to visit the website about communication with people with dementia on "A Place for Mom" at https://tinyurl.com/y32tccyd.

Independence

One of the hardest things about being diagnosed with dementia is the feeling of powerlessness. It is hard not to be able to manage life on your own. Learning to cope with dementia can be a great challenge.

Dementia diseases affect one's independence and quality of life. Below we have gathered some advice and products that can improve your quality of life despite dementia.

Memory systems

There is no definitive dividing line between common forgetfulness and memory problems in the early stages of dementia when the person starts having difficulties remembering names of things in the home, names of people they have known all their life, where they have placed the remote control, and so on.

Therefore, it's a good idea to introduce different memory systems into your daily routine, even if you may not need them yet. The reason is that the longer you have used them, the more natural the habit becomes and the longer it will persist and help you as the disease progresses.

Memory systems can be many things but they are all helpful in solving some of the challenges you face. It could be as simple as yellow post-its notes around the home, shopping lists, notes on the things to do or something completely different—or it could be some of the gadgets mentioned below.

Electronic calendars

Electronic calendars can help you remember. They can, for example, consist of electronic clocks or calendars that keep track of daily appointments and activities. Many such systems can do much more than a regular calendar.

For example, they can show pictures and tell you about daily tasks like vacuuming, having guests coming over for coffee, or sounding an alarm that tells you when to do something specific.

So, it is not just a calendar that you have to keep an eye on, but a tool that actively helps you remember what you need to achieve every day.

Medicine dispenser and medicine reminders

Electronic calendars, like medicine dispensers and medicine reminders, can also be considered 'reminder systems.' They help you get the right amount of medication at the right times of the day, so you get the treatment you need.

There are several types of medicine dispensers and they can do different things. What features you need depends, among other things, on how advanced the dementia is, whether you live alone, and whether you get help from caregivers. Therefore, research the market and see what you need before you buy a dispenser yourself.

Stay in touch

It is not easy to stay in touch when you get dementia and communication becomes a challenge, but it's important not to isolate yourself.

It is important to have a good social life. If you do not talk with people around you, you might feel lonely, and your quality of life will decline. If you want to keep going, be sure to stay in touch.

There are many ways to do so. It could be getting visits, going for walks with an acquaintance, or making phone calls. In recent years, there have been more and more opportunities for people with mild to moderate dementia to keep in touch with the outside world. Using ZOOM, Skype Wonder.me offer visual contact in addition to just voice connection. They can be set up in your electronic calendar (if you use oner), so you don't have to look up the web address every time.

Some solutions are created as part of your mobile phone. They are designed to be easy to use and get used to. In addition, there are also apps that remind you to call people around you.

Live 'dementia-friendly'

Most of us want to to be independent in our own home and manage our life on our own for as long as possible. In order for this to be possible, it may be an idea to make some changes to your home. Too many things and options can stress you out. Read the article in Section 2, p. 32 on what it means to live dementia-friendly and why it is important to think about.

Security alarms

It is estimated that half of all people who have dementia disappear for a shorter or longer period of time at some point.

Different technologies can help prevent this problem. GPS based tracking systems are very useful so others can keep an eye on where you are. Likewise, security alarms and fall alarms can help give you and your relatives a sense of security, both when you are at home alone or out of the house.

Both types of alarms can keep an eye on how you move around. Should anything happen to you, the alarm will call for help.

Information about such products can be found on the Internet.

Source:
Karger International: www.karger.com/Article/Pdf/333812

SECTION 3: LIFESTYLE ISSUES

CONTENTS

1.	Risk of dementia	page 48
2.	Diets	page 50
3.	The Mediterranean Diet	page 54
4.	Olive oil	page 57
5.	Exercise and dementia	page 60
6.	Exercise as a lifestyle	page 63
7.	Exercise - 5 good pieces of advice	page 66
8.	Exercise - get started	page 68
9.	Exercise without exercising	page 71
10.	Overweight	page 74
11.	Weight loss	page 76
12.	Sleep	page 78
13.	Dehydration	page 82

Risk of dementia

We all have some risk of dementia. Since dementia is a serious (and incurable) disease in all its forms, we must do what we can to reduce our risk of getting the disease. We start this Section with a summary of the factors that play a role in the development of dementia. In the following 12 articles, we dive deeper into them.

Risk and remedy

There are a number of things we can do to reduce the risk of dementia. Twelve critical, mid-life risk factors are listed below - nine are the original, well-known ones (Lancet Commission, 2017) and three (in italics) were added in 2020. Together, they make up approx. *40% of the causes of all dementia cases* (note: It is at best speculative if the causes of the other 60% are all to be found in our biology).

These known causes are (in relative order of importance; note: two share the 3rd and the 5th ranking):

Behavioral factors	Biological Factors	Social factors
3. *Concussions*	1. Hearing loss	2. Low education
3. Smoking	6. Hypertension	4. Depression
5. Exercise (lack of)	7. Diabetes	5. Social isolation
9. *Alcohol usage*		8. *Air pollution*
10. Overweight		

Interestingly, unlike the American Heart Association (see note below), the Lancet does not include *sleep* as a risk factor (and no explanation as to why not). Chronic sleep deprivation is mentioned by many researchers as one of the *most* important factors for good brain function and for increasing the risk of dementia, so we have added an article about sleep in this Section.

What should we do?

It is the general consensus that everyone can do something about most or all of these risk areas. Sure, it takes discipline to change your lifestyle. Go over the list again and think through each of the areas and see where you can make changes. Start with those that are the easiest for you.

Pollution may be an area that is not so obvious, but we can always find ways to limit our exposure to smoky and dusty environments, if nothing else, by limiting our time in polluted areas.

When should I start?

It cannot be said often enough, that whether you are young (under 45), middle-aged (45-65), or older (over 65), *now* is the time to start. It is never too late to improve your lifestyle, and given the alternative, it is far too serious to postpone it.

Start as early in life as possible with these factors. It is NOW to start, not in a week or a month, or a few years . . . or when you one day get time.

###

Note on sleep: AHA mentions in its reports that poor sleep, which can result from various sleep disorders, also has ties to different forms of cognitive decline. Experts state that many observational studies have confirmed this association, giving the example of research showing that insomnia can contribute to vascular dementia.

Sources:

Brain Health: Brain Institute at the University of Alabama at Birmingham School of Medicine reported in Medicalnewstoday.com: tinyurl.com/54pxte9a

The Lancet 2020, Vol 396, Issue 10248, p. 413ff - https://tinyurl.com/y6r25eqw

PS: The Lancet is one of the leading medical journals in the world. The Lancet Commission consists of 28 researchers from around the world. It publishes reports on all major health issues.

Diets

Usually, when we talk about healthy diets we think of our overall health and well-being. But new research shows that we in regards to brain health and dementia should be aware of the importance of diets.

The list of good advice is long. But what do we really know about what is good for brain health and brain functions? Well, one thing we are beginning to understand is how important healthy diet plans are for increasing the chance of delaying or preventing dementia and Alzheimer's.

The top 3 most important tips

1. Start the day with a healthy breakfast
A healthy brain starts with breakfast. Studies have found that breakfast improves short-term memory and attention. Students who eat breakfast every day score better on tests than those who do not. Do not skip it, even when you are late.

Healthy breakfast includes whole grain products (high in fiber), dairy products (with calcium), and fruit/berries (with vitamin C). Men should have 1 oz of fiber per day; women about 0.6 oz. But remember that twice as much is not twice as good. It has been found that a high calorie breakfast actually impedes concentration.

2. Include fish—the real brain food—in your diet
Fish, in particular fatty fish such as salmon, trout, tuna, mackerel, and sardines contain - in addition to valuable proteins - omega-3 fatty acids and DHA which are known to be absolutely essential for brain health. A diet that includes fatty fish twice a week has been linked to a lower risk of Alzheimer's and a general decline in brain function.

It is also believed that omega-3 containing diets increase memory capacity. Of all the diet groups mentioned here, fatty fish is the most important. If you wish, use spices instead of salt to give a fish dish some extra flavor. Turmeric is known to protect against Alzheimer's.

3. Get lots of blueberries—the superstar in the diet groups

Numerous animal experiments have shown that blueberries protect the brain from damage caused by free radicals. Polyphenols protect/prevent inflammation in the body, and reduce damage to our DNA. They have a positive effect on age-related disorders such as Alzheimer's and dementia. Experiments have shown that rats given blueberries have a cognitive function similar to much younger rats. Other studies confirm blueberries are important for learning and for muscle function. Eat them raw - in yogurt or salads - but remember that baking reduces the polyphenol content!

Three other important pieces of advice

4. Make avocados and whole grain part of your diet

All our organs are dependent on an abundant blood flow, but this is especially important for heart and brain function. A diet that contains abundant amounts of fruits, such as avocados, lowers the harmful L-cholesterol in the blood. L-cholesterol is responsible for the buildup of plaque and, consequently, decreased blood flow. And that is the cause of heart disease and, in the long run, dementia.

Avocados are a tasty and easy way to keep brain cells in order. Although they contain fats, they are the good mono-unsaturated fatty acids that promote blood flow. Use ripe avocados as a substitute for butter on the bread. Be prepared for a positive surprise! Eat plenty of whole grain products, but do not stop at whole grain breads. There are important B6 and B12 vitamins in whole grains that the brain needs. Quinoa and couscous are good substitutes for rice. Whole grains also protect against cancer and diabetes.

5. Remember a daily dose of *dark* chocolate and nuts

It will delight everyone with a sweet tooth to hear that *dark* chocolate (more than 70% cocoa) has a powerful antioxidant effect. Antioxidants prevent the harmful effect of free radicals in the body and brain. Chocolate also contains stimulating caffeine. Nuts and seeds are good sources of vitamin E, which also have antioxidant effect.

Research shows that these groups protect against impaired cognitive functions and dementia. Eat plenty of almonds, walnuts, Brazil nuts, cashews, pecans, flaxseed, and pistachios. They are all perfect as a snack in the morning or afternoon. Enjoy approx. 1 oz of nuts and dark chocolate a day. You get all the benefits without too many calories, fat, and sugar.

6. Don't forget to drink . . . water

We often do not think at all that water is one of the most important ingredients for a healthy life. In fact, the importance of water for both physical health and for brain functions cannot be overemphasized.

Most people know that you can survive without eating for a long time, *as long as you get water*. Water is critical for all the body's biological functions and invaluable for brain function.

Water helps "lubricate" the joints and regulate body temperature - and it is good for mood and well-being.

The rule of thumb is that if you are thirsty or your urine is darker than pale yellow, you're *already* dehydrated!

The body loses water all the time, even when we're not sweating. It happens during breathing. We breathe in relatively dry air, and exhale moist air with each breath. Particularly in cold weather! If we exercise or stay in a dry climate, the need for water is even greater.

Do not underestimate it; drink 6-8 glasses @ 8 oz a day. That sounds like a lot. Actually it's not; it becomes a habit - and an important one. If you need flavor in the water, you can use a slice of lemon - or have you ever thought about a slice of cucumber? You will be surprised there, too.

Coffee and alcohol are examples of drinks that *increase fluid loss* in the body, so enjoy both with caution.

Speaking about water and "fluid balance," read the article *Dehydration - or was it dementia* in Section 4, p. 82, and avoid a serious scare!

Source: The Lancet 2020, Vol 396, Issue 10248, p. 413ff - https://tinyurl.com/y6r25eqw

The Mediterranean Diet

No one talks about dementia and the Mediterranean diet in the same context. They should, because there's an increasing number of scientific studies that suggest those two subjects are related.

The Mediterranean diet contains all the ingredients that we now know with great certainty are important for our general health, cardiovascular functions, and so on.

But research is bringing a steady stream of articles showing the importance of these ingredients for memory and impaired brain function such as dementia/Alzheimer's.

The purpose here is to give you a quick overview of what the Mediterranean diet plan comprises—but also what food products you should stay away from as much as possible.

So, in short. . . **The Mediterranean diet** is based on the following food groups:
- vegetables, fruits, legumes, and whole grains
- healthy fats, such as nuts, seeds, and extra virgin olive oil
- moderate amounts of dairy products and fish
- very little white and red meat
- few eggs
- Turmeric (a superstar among spices when it comes to brain health)
- red wine in limited quantities
- plenty of water

And remember that the craving for sweets can be satisfied with dark (70%+) chocolate - *instead of* sugar-rich desserts!

In-between meals

Eating between meals is a temptation to eat sweets, empty calories, etc., so it is worth paying attention to the healthy *alternatives* recommended in the Mediterranean diet:
- small portions of nuts
- whole, fresh fruits (oranges, plums, grapes)
- dried fruits (apricots, figs)
- small portions of yogurt
- hummus with celery, carrots, other vegetables
- ripe avocados on whole wheat bread

What should you avoid?

Of course, there are food groups one must limit or completely avoid to ensure that the benefits gained from following the Mediterranean diet are not wasted.

It is recommended to avoid:
- processed cereal products (wheat bread, white pasta, pizza bread based on wheat flour)
- refined oils, incl. canola oil and soybean oil
- foods with added sugar (especially bakery products, sweets, sodas)
- processed meat products, incl. deli food, sausages/hot dogs
- processed/ready-made food products (incl. ready-made dinners)

A special warning: The more sugar you eat, the faster you age!

Sugar is a main cause of obesity (40% of the U.S. population) and it raises the risk of diabetes, cancer and Alzheimer's. The average American eats about 17 teaspoons of added sugar per day, roughly twice the amount recommended for men and three times the recommended amount for women. Avoid it *everywhere* you can! Read the product labels when you buy products in the store.

Your body will thank you for it.

Two final comments

There are many other good diet plans, but the Mediterranean diet plan attracted attention because of the longevity of people in the Mediterranean area. Few plans are backed by the extensive research on the ingredients that characterize the products in the Mediterranean diet.

Many people think that you have to eat like a rabbit to be healthy. The Mediterranean diet is filling, tasty, and - what is important to many - very varied.

Unless one is a fanatical supporter of red meat, the Mediterranean diet is highly recommended . . . also for families with small or older children.

Make it a lifestyle!

Bon appetite !

For the curious For more information on ingredients research in the Mediterranean diet, please refer to:
Aging Cells: https://tinyurl.com/yywd86mm
and
Medical NewsToday: https://tinyurl.com/y3fvz7n7

Olive oil

"Dementia and olive oil? You are kidding me, right?"
This is the reaction of many when they hear about a link between dementia and olive oil. We always think of low cholesterol and protection against heart disease when we think about olive oil. And for good reasons.

Below are the 'facts behind the fact' that olive oil is very important for cardiovascular health, which in turn is one of the important factors in lowering the risks for dementia.

In general, new research shows that olive oil may be the way to prevent dementia and Alzheimer's.

Olive oil is not just olive oil (see Note 1, below). In this article, we refer to "extra virgin olive oil" (or "EVOO") when we say "olive oil."

EVOO is high in mono-unsaturated fatty acids, which are the ones that protect against heart disease. But EVOO also has a high content of polyphenols, which are potent antioxidants.

Antioxidants have a major impact on our cognitive abilities (memory and focus) and can protect our brain cells from harmful substances. At least in mice.

Mice are, of course, not humans, but because mice for many decades have proven to be a good "model" for humans, this is where science begins.

And positive results in mouse experiments are always followed by human experiments. So it is worth noting the results from trials between 2012 and now.

Research results

These experiments showed that learning and memory (the ability to repeat learned skills) were improved when mice ate a diet rich in olive oil. They also showed evidence that olive oil could stop the negative effect of aging and impairment of cognitive abilities.

These experiments are all the more interesting because the mice were genetically modified in advance to have the three main characteristics of Alzheimer's (memory loss, beta amyloid buildup and tau protein—see Note 2 and 3 below). The researchers have concluded that there are two reasons for this improvement:

First of all, healthy "synapses" (the spaces between the brain cells, which control the communication of impulses from one cell to the next) are preserved.

The second reason is that the breakdown of brain cells is stopped and that the toxic waste products between the cells are removed.

The overall result is healthy synapses and good, fast, and consistant communication between the brain cells, which means good cognitive abilities.

So yes! It certainly seems to be fact and not fiction.

The future

Leading researchers believe that these two effects are crucial for the postponement of and possibly protection against the onset of dementia and Alzheimer's.

The next step is to see if EVOO can reduce dementia/Alzheimer's symptoms. The latter is important because affected people only come into treatment when the dementia condition already has started or is advanced.

Therefore, the possibility of reducing the conditions will be a big step on the way to a treatment of dementia/Alzheimer's. Olive oil seems to be a promising insurance against the deterioration of our brain functions as we age.

Until then . . .

. . . it is highly recommended to include the olive oil rich Mediterranean diet in your lifestyle.

In addition, it is recommended that, if you have the choice, buy only extra virgin olive oil. It is good for your general health, but it also seems to be a promising insurance against the deterioration of our brain functions as we get older.

NOTES

Note 1:

(a) "extra virgin" is the first 'press' (or squeeze out) of the oil;

(b) "virgin," is the second, and more powerful 'press;' and

(c) ordinary olive oil is extracted with solvents after the first two presses (the solvents are, of course, removed afterwards).

Note 2:

Amyloids form "plaque" (similar to what we know from our teeth) *between* the brain cells, preventing the communication that is the prerequisite for all brain activity.

Note 3:

Tau-protein helps with the transport of nutrients to the brain. However, in patients with Alzheimer's, this protein is trapped and accumulated *inside* the nerve cells, which die because they can no longer get the necessary nutrition.

Sources:
Aging Cells: https://tinyurl.com/yywd86mm
Medical NewsToday: https://tinyurl.com/y3fvz7n7

Exercise and dementia

There have not been many studies that show *why* the brain works better when we exercise. The reason for that is simple. Until recently, the technology has not been good enough to study the "mechanisms."

But we have long known exercise is an important factor in brain health. In this and the following three articles, we take a closer look at that.

In a fascinating article, a psychology professor at Northeastern University in Boston explains what is at stake. He has spent decades studying exercise and brain functions like focus, memory, and visual orientation. Below are the main conclusions from his article.

What *are* the mechanisms?
Brain cells (neurons) communicate by electrical impulses. When they work synchronously, it's like the spectators at a football game cheering at the same time when a team scores. These synchronous pulsations are what we call brain waves.

Low-frequency brain waves are characteristic of mundane, routine activities such as toothbrushing, driving, and sleeping. High-frequency waves, the so-called beta waves, are active when we are mentally engaged in activities that include memory, focus, and information processing, and brain waves are even more active when we exercise.

What happens when we exercise?
With aerobic exercise, our heart rate rises and our breathing becomes faster, the lungs supply the blood with more oxygen, and like the muscles, the brain absorbs more glucose and other carbohydrates.

But for a long time it was not clear what the brain used all that energy for.

Now it is known that the brain builds more neurotransmitters, i.e. more brain cell connections. . . and it is this renewal of the brain that is such an important result of exercising.

During exercise, the frequency and size of our brain waves change. We have more beta waves - that is, we are more "on our toes," more receptive to incoming information, especially visually stimulated information. It is important to be able to zoom in on things in the environment that may be critical to us - just like in the past, when you were either the "hunter" or the "prey" - and filter out the information that is not important.

So, do you get a younger brain?

Actually, yes, that's what it looks like!

First, studies show that exercise increases the production of growth promoters, which nourish new neurons and help existing cells to survive. New cells need more nourishment, and exercise is a way to provide them with what they need.

Second, there is a growth in the blood vessels that transport the nutrients. These changes come after a few weeks of exercise, but the effect lasts for a long time. The good thing is that the changes occur in the regions of the brain that are responsible for cognitive functions (the hippocampus). In other words, one gets a "younger" brain in terms of memory, concentration, multi-tasking, and processing of sensory impressions.

It has also been established that the gray brain mass grows when you exercise - and this is also in the regions that controls concentration and problem-solving abilities (general IQ).

All in all, these characteristics point to a brain that neurologists call "young brains."

Is exercise the magic solution?

While we should not expect a higher IQ by simply exercising, there is every reason to include even moderate exercise in one's lifestyle. Our health, and to a large extent our mental health, depends on whether we exercise or not.

One can even hope that many of our *physical* health problems also can be solved with exercise instead of medication. And if exercise does not sound so appealing, if the weather becomes a good excuse, etc., then remember that exercise does not have to be on a treadmill or outdoors. If the years of active sports are over, it's good to know that sex ranks on par with a 2 mi (3 km) brisk walk!

Sources for the curious:
Brain Health: Brain Institute at the University of Alabama at Birmingham School of Medicine reported in Medicalnewstoday.com: tinyurl.com/54pxte9a

The Lancet 2020, Vol 396, Issue 10248, p. 413ff - https://tinyurl.com/y6r25eqw

North Eastern University, Pennsylvania: https://tinyurl.com/y3bd7kqo
Journal of Neuroscience: http://www.jneurosci.org/content/36/8/2449

Exercise as a lifestyle

Exercise has been in the spotlight for many years, as one of the most important lifestyle factors for good health . . . for good reasons. There is increasing evidence that exercise is also important for brain health.

We therefore focus on this topic in four articles in this Section, partly because it is so important, and partly because it is a lifestyle factor that we can completely control ourselves - *even* **when physical obstacles seem to stand in the way.**

A healthy lifestyle, ranging from non-smoking and limited alcohol intake to healthy diet and weight control, is important for the prevention, postponement, and reduction of the effects of dementia.

The World Health Organization (WHO) has made it very clear that they consider exercise to be one of the most important lifestyle factors.

Why that is and what an individual can do to improve their situation is explained below.

Initially, it should be mentioned that the WHO estimates that citizens in the United States alone spend more than $2-3 Bn a year on popular memory apps. Unfortunately, there is not much to suggest they live up to the hope of a quick and easy memory improvement. WHO stresses it is much better to spend time exercising. That does not mean one should drop brain-teasers like crossword puzzles, Sudoku, and similar 'games.' They are useful - and are good entertainment.

Research-based recommendations

WHO says you should do 150 minutes of moderate physical activity per week. That is half an hour, 5 days a week (or 35-40 minutes 4 times a week). Aerobic activities that have a clear, positive connection to improved memory are bicycling, brisk walking, jogging, and swimming, as well as strength/weight training and tai chi. In other words, these are not *athletic* training programs that only a few can perform.

For the record, it cannot be ruled out that the "link" between memory and physical activity reflects the possibility that people who are motivated to exercise might have other characteristics (including genetic), which also has a positive influence on memory.

Why is exercise so good for the brain?

All exercise activities are good because they stimulates blood flow in the brain. It reduces the likelihood of getting what is called vascular dementia - a common form of dementia.

Physical activity also stimulates the formation of new blood vessels in the brain, which in turn contributes to better blood flow. And it is the increased blood flow that is important for the removal of harmful metabolic products that accumulate the brain.

Exercise also reduces the risk of high blood pressure and Type 2 diabetes. If you already have either one of them, exercise can help reduce the severity. Keep in mind that both of these disorders are in themselves associated with dementia.

Finally, exercise can both prevent and relieve depression, and help to achieve better sleep, both of which are also risk factors for dementia.

A major study

A rare long-term study on dementia and exercise was published in 2017. It started in 1985 and included more than 3,200 adults aged 18 to 30 years. When it ended, the subjects were in their mid-50s. The study showed that people who watched TV for more than 3 hours a day or otherwise failed to exercise regularly, even moderately, had impaired mental function and slower brain activity later on in life.

It's worth making a mental note on that—or even better, *Change!*

Exercise is a shortcut to social living

Another important aspect of exercise is that people who are physically active usually have several social activities that require mental commitment. It can be anything from a jogging club and adult football to basketball pickup, ballroom dancing, and doubles tennis. Activities with intellectual stimulation, such as a book club, bridge, or discussion forum, are also important.

Together, contrary to sitting in front of the TV, these social activities help to make us mentally active and healthy. Remember, although it is best to start before seeing the first signs of dementia, *it's never too late to start*.

So, start NOW! Make exercise a part of your daily routine.

Note:

This article is based on information from the Mount Sinai School of Medicine in New York, V.A. Boston Healthcare System, Boston University's School of Public Health, and Harvard T.H. Chan School of Public Health

Sources:

For the curious: To read about exercise and cognitive function, see article in Psychiatry, 2017: https://tinyurl.com/y363cvmr.

Getting around - 5 good pieces of advice

You know exercise and moving around are good for your health, but you may not feel you have the time or energy to engage in club life or fit regular training times into everyday life. The good thing is that it does not have to be time consuming or cumbersome.

Physical activity in everyday life can seem to be too time consuming, but it does not have to be that way. It's all starts by making it become a natural part of your daily chores. You are already moving during the day, and often only small adjustments are needed to optimize your exercise and strengthen the body.

Here are 5 tips on how to include exercise and movement into everyday activities:

1. Use the stairs

Use the stairs whenever you have the opportunity, like in the shopping malls, in office buildings, and, if you live in multi-story apartment buildings. Maybe you can start by using the stairs half the way; and you don't have to walk up very fast. Stair-stepping is good for overall fitness, aerobic fitness, but particularly for the leg muscles.

2. Get off the bus one stop early

If you take the bus to and from work or a trip to the city because it is too far to walk, consider getting off the bus stop earlier than usual. It may be just what it takes to increase your heart rate that day, and that is always healthy for the heart and the circulation!

3. Set the pace for cleaning and gardening

Whatever the season, the home must be cleaned and the garden must be cared for. When the floors need to be scrubbed, the windows need to be washed, and the flower beds need to be trimmed, then put a serious effort into it and break a sweat on the forehead. It all strengthens your muscles.

4. "Active" TV-watching

Many people sit back comfortably on the couch when watching TV, but you should consider making TV-watching into an activity of higher intensity. For example, if you have an exercise bike, a Nordic Track, or a yoga mat that you put away and are now collecting dust, pull it in front of the television. It could very well be that your favorite program takes *away* the focus on the hard work of exercising.

5. Put music on the system and dance

Make sure to make room in your home for you to move around. Then put your favorite CD on the system and dance! If you have a partner, pull him or her up from the chair for a swing. Dancing makes both the pulse and the mood rise.

You will enjoy how you feel!

Exercise - Let's get started!

So, you have actually thought that you would like to start exercising, but you don't quite know 'where' to start. Does that ring a bell?

But 'not knowing where to start' is a bad, yet common, excuse for 'not doing.'

Read on and get good advice on how to start having a more active lifestyle.

In general, there's a lot of focus in our society on healthy, active bodies - and for good reasons. Regular exercise is crucial for maintaining a good health and coping well in life - and on top of it, it's considered the best medicine for preventing falling!

Although we do believe physical activity in general is good, it is not always enough for us to change our behavior and start exercising. There are many ways to be physically active, but it can be difficult to figure out what kind of activity to choose and how to get started.

We will help you with that here.

It's joyous to do it together

. . . and it's also much easier to get out and start training when you're two or more. When physical activity is on the program, it can be hard to get off of the couch; if you "cancel," it doesn't affect anyone other than yourself . . . but if you have a training partner, then someone is counting on you, and then it's much harder to cancel.

Ask your spouse, neighbor, friend or an acquaintant if you should start an activity together. Or ask someone you know who is already involved in an activity you are interested in, if you can tag along next time they go. Conversely, if it is you who is already active, then see if there's someone in your circle of friends who would like to join you.

Find an exercise that suits you

Consider who you are and what you like. Are you a competitive person? Do you prefer to stay indoors or outdoors? What matters to you? Do you like to immerse yourself in only one thing - alone? Take time to think about this, and then use your considerations to choose your type of exercise.

First of all, it is important to find an exercise form you like. If you do not think it is fun to exercise, it will be a struggle to get started or keep going. And in the worst case scenario, you end up not going at all.

Don't forget, though, that ordinary daily activities such as gardening, vacuuming, stair climbing, and the walk to the grocery store *also* count as physical activity.

Get help finding activities near you

Maybe you already know which activity you want to embark on. Maybe you're open to trying all sports as long as it takes place with others *in your age group*. Whatever you are looking for, there are plenty of websites based on zip code, city, sport, age group, and gender. That makes it easy to find the activity that suits you.

When you click on the various pin markings on the map, the associations' contact information appears. At the same time, you can see if the associations offer activities for your age group and gender.

Training by yourself

If you would rather train alone, you can use tools that will make it easier for you to get started.

Many apps have been developed for the mobile phone or iPad. They help you train by yourself or with a nursing home helper. You can also get tailor-made training programs that suit your specific challenges and physical needs. Many apps have a training diary so you can keep track of your progress.

Timers

There are also timers that can help you with interval training, which is especially good for the heart and circulation. You can use them to control your workout, whether you are running or walking. They are easy to use, and you can put together a complex training program without having to enter a single number. Many have a "Play" button, which starts a simple interval training and continues until you stop it yourself.

Pedometers

If you are not ready for a more committed exercise, walking is the perfect way to start. Walking counteracts depression, strengthens your brain, your heart, and your muscles and bones. And walking is gentle on your joints.

Do yourself a favor and buy a pedometer! By using it, you get a clear insight into how much you move during a day. It is motivating to know that even taking the trash out is a bit of exercise.

With a pedometer, you can also set a goal for how many steps you want to walk in a day. The pedometer constantly shows you how many steps are left until you reach the goal of the day. That's good for motivation. Studies show that pedometers actually make us move more, so just get started!

Another thought . . .

Many people think it can be difficult to find the time to exercise regularly, but there is help to be found in the article *Exercise - 5 good pieces of advice,* p. 66.

Sources:
Move for life: https://www.bevaegdigforlivet.dk/
JAMA Network: https://tinyurl.com/y38rta3o

Exercise without exercising

If you have read the four previous articles about exercising, you might already be tired and think, wouldn't it be great if you had a pill that could reduce the risk or prevent dementia from developing the same way exercise can - but without exercising?

Well, some research actually suggests that *exercise without exercising* is a way to a better brain.

1. Exercise is good for health

Significant material already exists which shows that exercise is important for the body. It is also known that exercise increases the formation of new neurons in the brain and stimulates learning and memory in both younger and older people. There is even talk of protecting the functions of the brain against the reduction that comes with age.

But we don't know much about what happens at the actual cell level in the brain when you exercise. This is the focus of the latest research.

2. Exercise has an effect on the cells in the brain

Here are five points to consider.

- Exercise initiates a cascade reaction of substances in the brain - substances we don't know a whole lot about. These substances react with and initiate other processes, which ultimately have an effect on how the brain works. The reason for the lack of knowledge is, among other things, that previous studies focused on transferring blood from mice that exercised to mice that did not. The latter group achieved better brain function, but this raised the question of whether it was exercise or the "young" blood that had the positive effect.

- In new studies, young and older mice exercised for six weeks. The blood from both groups was then transferred to a group of non-exercising mice. These mice got better brain function, whether they got blood from the young or the older exercising mice. That precludes that age plays a role. It's the actual exercise that matters!
- With renewed curiosity, the researchers then examined what the difference in the blood of the exercising and non-exercising mice was. They found a large number of proteins that were not present in non-exercising mice. Of particular interest is a small protein (called GPLD1), which is produced in the liver - an organ that has not previously been linked to brain function.
- Finally, the researchers used genetic engineering to increase GPLD1 production in the liver from older, non-exercising mice. These mice now functioned just as well as young mice in terms of learning and memory. The older mice also produced many more new neurons. In other words, they worked just as well as the mice that exercised.
- Encouraged by this, experiments were carried out on older men and women, and - long story short - the result was the same! Exercise increases GPLD1 when exercising! And GPLD1 is good for brain functions.

3. Get som exercise without exercising

Based on these experiments and on the fact that we now know more about which substances act on the brain's functions, and given that we can now also produce these substances in the laboratory, it is tempting to conclude that now you can just take GPLD1 and preserve and improve learning and memory - *without exercising*.

Voila!

And while this probably *is* true, it should be emphasized that there are many important *physiological* benefits to exercising (see, for example, the two special articles mentioned below). But for those people who, for various reasons *cannot* exercise - and there are many of them in the older age group - these results are very encouraging.

That's a topic we'll hear more about in the future.

Sources:

This article is based on material from the University of California, San Francisco and a report from it published in the journal Science (https://science.sciencemag.org/content/369/6500/167).

See the four other exercise articles in this Section, above.

Overweight

We talk a lot about being overweight but never about the possible impact of overweight on dementia. We should, though, because new research shows a connection even *before* we get "old."

There is no shortage of good suggestions for losing weight, and although we know it is important, it is often difficult to maintain the motivation to do something about it (we did not say anything about broken New Year's resolutions). If you need a new motivation, here it is:

Being overweight in your younger years carries an increased risk of dementia later in life.

A large number of studies indicate that obesity early in life (20-49 years) is a risk factor for dementia later in life. And the brutal fact is that when dementia strikes, it's too late to reverse the negative trend in the cognitive functions - although it's always healthy to lose weight. . . and never too late to start.

New research
Published results are based on the so-called Body Mass Index - BMI (see below) and the age groups were divided into three:
(1) early adulthood (20-49)
(2) middle ages (50-69) and
(3) older (70-89).

The results of these studies provide a varied picture of the link between obesity and dementia. There are differences between gender and age as well as many other health factors . . . but the researchers nonetheless point out that obesity in early adulthood (20-49 years) carries a 30-50% increased risk of dementia after 70 years. The results also raise the question of whether (1) obesity in younger years inevitably leads to dementia and (2) whether weight loss through exercise can prevent it? So there will be a focus on these topics in the coming years.

What can you do?
Unfortunately, this is not yet known, so the researchers point to the lifestyle factors we know a lot about and always talk about, diet and exercise. The earlier in life you start with good eating habits, exercise, etc. (see articles about this, starting p. 75 in), the better are the chances of preventing or delaying dementia.

REMEMBER that in all "public health studies," it is important to distinguish between a 'link' or 'connection' as something different from 'a cause.' In other words, these results do not conclude that obesity *causes* dementia, only that dementia occurs more frequently in people who were overweight as adolescents and during mid-life, and that obesity therefore is called an important risk factor.

Definition: BMI (Body Mass Index) expresses body fat in relation to height and weight. It is calculated as weight (in kg) divided by the square of height (in meters) - BMI is an approximate calculation.
The BMI categories are:
   Underweight: <18.5
   Normal weight: 18.5–24.9
   Overweight: 25–29.9
   Obesity> 30
Example: A man who weighs 176 lbs (80 kg) and is 6 ft tall (180 cm or 1.8 m) has a BMI of 24.6. If he weighs 198 lbs (90 kg) he is overweight and if he weighs more than 220 lbs (100 kg) he is obese. See also the article *Weight Loss* on the next pages.

Source:
See also: The Lancet 2020, Vol 396, Issue 10248, p. 413 - https://tinyurl.com/y6r25eqw
Risk of dementia WebMD article: - https://tinyurl.com/y47ky3pc

Weight loss

If you are a relative of a person with dementia, you have most likely experienced that meals can be an almost insurmountable challenge. Weight loss is almost inevitable. If you provide support and peace of mind, there is a greater chance of maintaining appetite and avoiding weight loss in people with dementia.

Why do you stop eating?

Almost all people with dementia experience weight loss. Often it is related to the fact that the person with dementia forgets to eat, no longer feels hungry, or may not be able to understand why one should eat. This, of course, has to do with how advanced dementia is.

Besides the fact that people with dementia can forget when and why they should eat, they can also forget how. Even using a knife and fork can become a challenge at some point.

Remind the person with dementia about the meals

There are very easy ways to get people with mild dementia to eat.

Often it's enough to remind them of it and then he or she will find it reasonably natural to eat. This is true even if they are not aware that they are hungry.

But you may not always be around, so if you want to help the person to eat, you can invest in assistive devices.

In such cases, an electronic calendar or other types of memory systems can be a good solution (p. 36).

Memory systems can help make a person with dementia independent for a longer period of time and increase their quality of life.

Help with the food

Getting help to eat can have a big impact on how much people with dementia consume during a day. Depending on how far the disease has progressed, help with food can be several things. People who are in the early stages of dementia may need to be reminded that it's time for food. It may help them to watch you eat while having meal together.

People with advanced dementia may need to be reminded about what food is, why they should eat, or even have physical help to eat.

Support and peaceful surroundings are crucial to success

Caregivers point out that the physical and social *surroundings* of the meal is important.

Noisy, restless or unsafe surroundings can ruin the appetite, whereas a good and cozy atmosphere around the meal can help increase the desire to eat and even stimulate the appetite. Therefore, it can often pay off to allocate enough time to eat so the person will not feel stressed.

A word about alcohol and dementia

Most people know that alcohol has unwanted properties. This is why the National Board of Health recommends limited intake for healthy people (1 drink per day for women and 2 for men).

It can be more harmful for a person with dementia to drink alcohol than it is for a healthy person, because the function of the brain is already impaired. Therefore, a person with dementia is more affected by alcohol than a healthy person and should ideally avoid alcohol entirely.

Always talk **to your doctor** or other health professional if you have questions about eating habits or the diet for a person with dementia.

Sleep

Did you know that sleep is actually one of the most important factors for brain health? According to new research, getting enough sleep is critical to delaying or preventing dementia and Alzheimer's.

Not only that . . .

Research also shows *why* sleep is a critical factor. And that is not good news.

Sleep problems are very common. We used to think it was mostly elderly people who have sleep problems, but new studies have shown that many younger people who use social media at night time have serious anxiety problems (depression, low self-esteem, etc.) leading to sleep problems.

Many brain scientists call it "a national crisis." And even worse, one cannot compensate for the harmful effect of only five to six hours of sleep per night by taking an afternoon nap - regardless of how good it may feel.

The basics

We have several phases of sleep each night. First comes the light sleep. Several hours later comes the deep sleep, and finally comes the dream phase, the so-called REM phase (Rapid Eye Movement) - often right before we wake up. Each phase has its characteristic brain waves.

Researchers have in recent years determined that the brain cells turn on and off at different times during the day, but work in the same rhythm (synchronization) in the deep-sleep phase. When they are all "off," the brain does not need much oxygen.

This results in a reduced need for blood supply to the brain. This in turn allows slow waves of the fluid that surrounds the brain to flow out and take with it the toxins (including beta amyloid and tau protein) that have accumulated during the day.

And it is the accumulation of amyloid that can cause dementia and Alzheimer's.

Do not wait until you are older

We often hear how important a good night's sleep is for our health, good mood, cognitive functions (first and foremost memory), and our daily productivity. All that is correct.

But in our busy, stressful, and super-connected, online lives, many people say "we can sleep when we get old." The irony of that is that you will get there faster if you do *not* get enough sleep.

Besides, there's nothing to suggest that you even sleep *better* as you get older.

And if it was only energy and productivity that were challenged by lack of sleep, it would not be so bad with a few hours less.

The findings conclude . . .

But the latest research results demonstrate anew the importance of 7-8 hours of sleep. The main reason is that these slow in-and-out flows of cerebrospinal fluid only take place while we are in deep sleep. It is a phase we cannot control, and there are no shortcuts to reach this phase. We cannot shorten or skip phase 1; nor can we shorten sleep by avoiding the REM dream phase. In other words, there's no way around it. When it comes to sleep, 7-8 hours of sleep a night is the only way to good brain health.

Problems and solutions

Since you have no control over the sleep phases, what can you do to avoid the situation where "at night I cannot sleep; in the morning I cannot wake up!"

When you have a restless night and are constantly looking at the clock, one of the best things to do is to get up and go to another room, eat just a little bit, do things that are soothing, including reading, and possibly take a hot bath. When you feel the fatigue coming back, go to bed again.

To find out *why* you don't get the sleep you need, start with keeping a simple "sleep diary" for a week or two, recording bedtimes, how often you wake up, go to the bathroom, eating and exercise habits, etc. It can provide inspiration for changes in habits that are worth making.

What can you do?
- Often, irregular bedtimes is a cause. Change your habits.
- Eating too late at night can be a problem. Avoid eating and drinking approx. 4 hours before going to bed. Avoid strong spices, caffeine and alcohol in the evening. A drink or two can help you relax, but it does *not* give you a good night's sleep.
- Be aware that many types of medication can be a cause of sleep problems. It is worth considering whether to reduce the intake of medication, but only after consultation with your doctor.
- Avoid or limit TV and the use of computers/tablets right before bedtime or certainly not while in bed. The bluish screen light reduces melatonin, which is a sleep-inducing hormone
- If there is annoying noise in or around the home, you can use "white noise" to mask it. It can be, for example, a fan in the bedroom or "white noise music" (nature sounds from forest, beach or mountains).
- Get about 30 minutes of exercise most days of the week, even if it is relatively close to bedtime.

###

LATEST UPDATE
Very new reports conclude that if you constantly go to bed two hours later and get up at the usual time, you risk
- mental problems like reacting slowly
- impulsively making several mistakes

- generally worse mood and emotions
- anxiety and stress related problems and PTSD
- physical problems like developing Type-2 diabetes, cardiovascular diseases, and overweight.

Unfortunately, the development of the above mentioned problems is a two-way traffic. **Lack of sleep leads to problems, but those problems also lead to poorer and shorter sleep.** This is a self-reinforcing process that one must do everything to avoid - regardless of gender, age, lifestyle, and regardless of whether dementia is diagnosed or not.

It is not always easy to get enough sleep - *or at least we think so!*

But it's not a matter of "finding time" for enough sleep; it is a matter of "taking time" for enough sleep.

It's a lifestyle factor that we fortunately can do something about. Even if you don't like the idea of taking sleeping pills, it is a better alternative than getting on the slippery slope of sleep depravation. Alternatively, consider herbs or other natural sleep assisting products. Under all circumstances, talking to your doctor about sleeping pills is a good way to go.

Don't put it off until after the worst bustle is over, or when the big project is over, and certainly not until you get older. We never get enough time to handle it all.

A good night's sleep should be a very high priority!
Sleep well!

Sources:

Here is one of the most summarized groups of articles on sleep from Medical News Today: https://tinyurl.com/y4cxefyq

See also: The Lancet 2020, Vol 396, Issue 10248, p. 413ff - https://tinyurl.com/y6r25eqw and JAMA article: https://tinyurl.com/y4e6gfop; and for the really curious: Sleep and toxins in the brain: https://tinyurl.com/y2drr8w8.

Dehydration

Was it dementia or not?

That was the question for a 70-year-old man after three scary memory episodes that may be helpful for others to know about. Here's his personal story about them.

Growing concern

On a hot, humid summer morning in Miami, Florida in 2011, my wife and I were out for a bike ride in the neighborhood. When we got home and cooled off in the driveway, my wife could see that "something was wrong" with me. After a bit of mumbling, I embarrassedly asked if we were heading out on our bike ride or if we had just returned home.

After the initial scare had subsided, we went inside, drank fresh water, cooled off . . . and all the details from the bike ride came back. I could with full clarity tell where we had been, what we had seen, etc., and we dismissed the episode as "something strange."

But the same thing repeated itself a few months later. One morning when my wife came home from the post office, I got up from my desk and asked where she had been. We were on the verge of concluding that I had not listened properly to what she had told me, but when she with initial nervousness asked what I had done while she was away, I had no recollection of it.

We decided to go to the hospital, and already on the way over there all the details of that morning came back. At the hospital, no explanation could be found. When I spoke to my own doctor the following week, he referred to it as dehydration - a major problem for older people.

A few years later, we moved to Arizona and lived in a rented apartment before buying a house. One Saturday morning - after getting the keys to the house - my wife came home with a couple of our good friends to whom we wanted to show the house. I hesitated. I was confused. "Have we bought a house?" I asked. I had no recollection of that! Concern, embarrassment, and the feeling of loss emerged - again

But 15 minutes later, on the way over to the house, all the details about it came back, the address, who the seller was, the floor plan, the decor, etc.

Relief after check with doctor

We decided to seek advice from a neurologist. After an extensive series of tests and scans, the answer came back. There were no signs of dementia at all - "rather the opposite," said the neurologist.

The diagnosis was 'transient amnesia' or plainly, *temporary* lack of memory.

The characteristic is that only the short-term memory is affected and that it only lasts a few hours, and often much less. And the most important thing is that *the memory is not lost*. It is *inaccessible* for a shorter period of time! There is no medical explanation for the phenomenon, but the neurologist suggested "dehydration!"

The take-away is the following:

Seek advice in any situation that pertains to memory loss. It can be an incipient dementia - but it can also be something as innocent as lack of water (or lack of sleep, improperly adjusted medication, and other things). We must maintain the body's water balance - every day, *even if we do not exercise and/or sweat!*

We constantly exhale moist air and inhale air of far less humidity. The result is that dehydration sneaks up on you!

Do not make that mistake!

You can read more about transient memory loss, at Wikipedia: https://tinyurl.com/hefzxrz

SECTION 4: WORTH KNOWING - SPECIAL SUBJECTS

CONTENTS

1.	Blood test/Alzheimer's	page 86
2.	Blood pressure	page 88
3.	Pollution	page 92
4.	Better memory	page 94
5.	Immune system	page 97
6.	Inflammations	page 101
7.	L-serine	page 103
8.	Medical drugs - be careful!	page 105
9.	New medicine for Alzheimer's	page 107
10.	Medicine for dementia - do they work?	page 109
11.	Menopause	page 111
12.	Dizziness	page 114
13.	Tests or not	page 116
14.	Vaccination	page 119

Blood test for Alzheimer's

A blood test for Alzheimer's has not previously existed. But now a technique has been developed and tested in Sweden and the USA. Such a blood test for Alzheimer's is a major step towards an early diagnosis.

Today, the development of Alzheimer's is determined only *after* the symptoms appear in a person. This is because the diagnosis is based on memory tests, which are typically not started until the symptoms appear. And only then is the diagnosis confirmed using expensive PET brain scans. In other words, the disease may be advanced at the time the diagnosis is made.

The idea of a blood test is therefore not new. Unfortunately, previous methods, incl. samples taken from cerebrospinal fluid, have not lived up to expectations. It has therefore long been a desire to find a test that can determine early, easily, and reliably whether a person is at risk of getting Alzheimer's.

The blood test

The new test looks for small amounts of a protein called p-tau217, which researchers are quite sure is the factor that reduces and, over time, destroys memory and learning functions. It has now been proven that tau protein is found in the blood many years before the symptoms of the disease appear - according to one Swedish researcher, maybe as early as 20 years before.

The blood test is very simple, requires only 4 ml of blood, and can determine the presence of tau protein with 96% accuracy. This degree of simplicity makes the blood sample cheap and easy to be used widely.

Another interesting observation is that the blood test can distinguish between Alzheimer's and other degenerative brain diseases. So, there are good reasons to share the researchers' optimism that a much earlier diagnosis gives people at risk of

Alzheimer's opportunities to slow or maybe even prevent its development.

Can I have such a blood test now?

The test is still a lab-based test, and the method needs to be tried out in much larger numbers to determine its value; therefore, it cannot yet be used by your GP.

However, people with a family-based history of Alzheimer's case may enter studies even if they have not yet developed symptoms.

Is a blood test a good idea?

As you know, Alzheimer's can not yet be cured, and it raises the question of whether or not it's a good idea to get such a test when it soon becomes available. Although there is no doubt that a very early diagnosis has a number of advantages, it's not as straightforward as it sounds. We will refer to the arguments for and against an Alzheimer's test, p. 116.

Source:
JAMA article about the blood test: https://tinyurl.com/yydoxbxn.
Also read the article *Test or no test*, below.

Blood pressure

Did you know that high blood pressure is a risk factor for dementia and Alzheimer's?
Studies show it is a risk factor for brain tissue damage. Given how common high blood pressure is, this is a subject of intense research.

It has been known since the 1960s that high blood pressure increases the pressure on the body and leads to numerous ailments and diseases, and also leads to cognitive problems (such as impaired responsiveness in motorists and pilots).

But it is relatively new that higher than normal blood pressure over longer periods of time can have a negative impact on memory, attention span, and the speed at which the brain processes information.

High blood pressure is common

More than one-third of *all* people and about 80% of people over the age of 65 have high blood pressure. (blood pressure is explained in the footnote below). Given this large number of people, knowledge about the risks associated with high blood pressure is extremely important.

Our blood pressure changes with age. The scientific community points to the following reasons:
- changes in hormone profile
- narrowing of blood vessels (linked to cholesterol)
- more salt in the food (taste buds deteriorate with age, so we tend to use more of it)
- less efficient heart muscle

High blood pressure and the brain

Researchers in Chicago conducted a study of 1,300 elderly people to see if there was a direct link between high blood pressure and three critical, physical factors in the brain of the elderly:

- plaque - the buildup of tau protein between brain cells
- tangles, the distortion of the fiber structure inside the brain cells
- infarcts, "dead" areas of the brain caused by blockages of blood flow

The test persons were examined every year for the last years of their lives (an average of 8 years). Two-thirds had high blood pressure years before the trial started and 87% took blood pressure lowering medication. After they died, they were autopsied. It was found that half had at least one infarct.

Results

There was a 46% increase in the risk of brain damage if one had a 13 points higher systolic blood pressure (147 instead of 134). This damage was equivalent to having a nine years older brain.

The researchers then looked at the link between high blood pressure and the structure of brain cells in people with Alzheimer's.

Here the connection was less clear. Although there was a tendency for increased "tangles" in patients with high blood pressure, there was no clear tendency for increased plaque. Why the two phenomena do not go together is not known.

In another trial, it was demonstrated that if you have high blood pressure when you are in your 50s, you have a higher risk of getting dementia later in life.

What can you do?

First of all, it is important to keep an eye on your blood pressure. Check it at least once a year (a too low blood pressure should also be monitored; it can lead to other problems, incl. a tendency to fall and faint).

Fortunately, there are several things that counteract the influence of age on high blood pressure.

Here are the 6 easiest:
- To start with the simplest, take 6 deep breaths for 30 sec several times a day; the systolic blood pressure drops by 3 points
- Eat healthy and get exercise (see the five articles on *Lifestyle* starting on p.48). A diet rich in fruits and vegetables lowers blood pressure as much as many blood pressure lowering medical products on the market. A 30 minutes of moderate exercise a day (e.g. walking on an exercise belt) further lowers blood pressure
- Limit your intake of salt; this is critical. Most Americans consume way too much salt and not enough potassium, both of which negatively affect blood pressure. Avoid ready-made and processed foods - they have a high content of salt; limit your consumption of chips/snacks, ready-made soups, and dinner dishes
- Do hand-grip exercises! Surprisingly, research has shown that the use of a hand spring or clamp ball for 2 min at a time for a total of 14-15 minutes every other day, lowers blood pressure. No one knows why.
- Avoid medications used for colds as well as NSAIDs (non-steroidal, anti-inflammatory drugs), such as Advil and Motrin; they can raise blood pressure.
- And talk to your doctor about whether you may need to adjust your blood pressure lowering medication.

Notes:
Our blood pressure is expressed in millimeters of mercury (Hg) and consists of two numbers, *systolic* and *diastolic* blood pressure.

Systolic blood pressure is the high number and represents the maximum pressure in the heart chambers when the heart contracts and pushes the blood into the body's blood vessels.

The diastolic blood pressure is the low number and represents the pressure in the heart between heartbeats, i.e. while the heart fills up with blood again.

Blood pressure it typically measured with a cuff placed on the upper arm.

Important ranges:

A normal blood pressure is below 120/80 mm Hg - called "120 over 80," according to CDC, National Institute of Health, and American Heart Association (Nov. 2017 recommendations).

AHA also recommends that people with high blood pressure over 130/80 should receive treatment (stage I hypertension). Blood pressure higher than 140/90 is now called Stage II hypertension.

Keep an eye on your blood pressure: For every rise in blood pressure of 20/10 mm Hg, the risk of cardiovascular diseases doubles!

Sources:
Medical News - https://tinyurl.com/yyuevhwb
See also: The Lancet 2020, Vol 396, Issue 10248, p. 413ff - https://tinyurl.com/y6r25eqw
Journal of Neurology: https://tinyurl.com/y66smv29

Pollution

When we talk about risk factors for dementia, we normally talk about lifestyle factors. Nobody talks about pollution - until now . . .

While pollution (in this article we talk about *only* air pollution, but we will soon include microplastics) has long been associated with poor health, it has been overlooked as a factor in dementia. But new research strengthens a presumption that *air pollution* can lead to dementia and Alzheimer's.

One report even indicates that as many as 20% of all dementia cases are due to pollution. What is new in these reports is the discovery that the polluting air particles penetrate the body and change the brain. These changes are directly related to failing cognitive functions. With 45-50 million people with dementia worldwide and no cure in sight, it is a colossal problem and concern.

Size matters - small particles are the culprit

Other reports explains the underlying mechanism.

One study of more than 3,600 elderly women in the United States showed that a high level of particles with a diameter of *less than* 2.5μ (micro-meters) increases the risk of dementia by more than 92% compared to a contamination with particles greater than 2.5μ.

A similar, detailed experiment was conducted over a 15-year period in Sweden. The conclusion was the same. People exposed to contamination by very small particles have an increased risk of impaired cognitive functions.

These very small particles come from the combustion in power plants and from the exhaust from cars, and because the particles are so small and stay in the air for a long time, it is very difficult to avoid inhaling such particles. They end up in the brain and start making changes in the brain cells. According to the World Health

Organization, 90% of the world's population is exposed to air pollution, and several million people die each year as a direct result.

What can you do?

Pollution is particularly worrying because it is an area that we - apart from very limited actions in everyday life - can not do much about. Pollution is local, national and international. Pollution respects no boundaries. And we will live with it for many, many years. So what specifically *can* we do? Focus on lifestyle issues (Section 3, p. 47).

It's the best way - in fact the only way - to keep the brain healthy. *Do not postpone it!*

Sources:
Nature.com - https://tinyurl.com/y65pehv6
WHO - https://www.who.int/health-topics/air-pollution
British Journal of Medicine: https://tinyurl.com/yy7atpq6

Better memory

Wouldn't it be great if there was a method to improve your memory?

Well, there is. And it's easy, comfortable, and it works. As a matter of fact, you don't have to do anything - *literally!*

If you want a better memory, here's the easy way.

Take a break!

When we try to remember what we have learned, it is reasonable to assume that the more work we put into it, the better we become at remembering it. New research shows that the opposite is true. You can improve your memory by doing nothing at all. . . literally!

The memory of what is learned is preserved much better if you after learning something "take a break" of approx. 10 minutes of quiet thinking, perhaps meditation, perhaps with dimmed light, and without any interruptions or new activities.

In other words, we must avoid doing or thinking about all the small chores like checking emails, web surfing, texting, phone calls; they all interfere with the delicate process of memory formation.

Anyone can do it

It has great value for students, but anyone can benefit from this method. And it's worth emphasizing that people with impaired cognitive functions, incl. Alzheimer's also have positive results with this method.

It's actually a 120 year old discovery. Two German psychologists experimented around 1900 with "memory consolidation." They did this by having their students memorize meaningless word-syllables. Then, one half got another list of syllables, while the other half got a break of 6 minutes. After 90 minutes, all the students were tested. The group that had a break remembered twice as many of the syllables as the group that did not have a break. Our ability to remember is very fragile right after learning new information. It is easily disturbed by other new, incoming information. But it took more than 100 years before these observations were taken seriously.

New experiments confirm the method

Studies in England and the United States have since confirmed the original data. In new experiments, two groups of people *with incipient memory problems* were given a 15-word list. One of the groups then received other memory tests immediately after, while the other group was given a 10 min break in a dark room (without falling asleep). The group with "other activities" could remember 14% of the words while the "pause group" could remember 49% of the words, which is almost the same as in groups of people without memory problems.

A continuation of the experiments was even more surprising. Participants listened to a story and answered questions afterwards. Those who had no break could remember 7% of the details of the story. Those who had a break could remember 79% of the details! An improvement that was far greater than for completely healthy people (improvement of memory of up to 30%).

The conclusions are unanimous

All these studies have since been repeated. The conclusions (that apply to people with *and* without memory problems) are that a short break without any activity . . .
- improves the memory of details for both younger and older people
- improves memory of 3-dimensional facts (spatial orientation, landmark recognition, "where did I put my keys?" etc.)
- has a lasting effect

It is worth mentioning that post-trial questionnaires showed that most of the participants simply "let their minds wander," i.e. not thinking on anything in particular. Contrarily, any focus on a "topic" is a distraction. To avoid that, meditation is an extremely important component in improving memory.

It should be mentioned that researchers do not yet know why this "pause" has an effect on memory, but there are indications that newly formed learning (memory) must be cemented in long-term memory in order to become lasting.

It has always been thought that this 'cementing' happen during sleep, when the hippocampus communicates with the cerebral cortex, but this is obviously not the case or at least not the whole truth.

While researchers search for 'the whole truth,' the rest of us can rejoice in the fact that something as easy and relaxing as "doing nothing," can have such a positive effect.

And in that regard, we should "remember," that in an age of an abundance of information and incessant interruptions, a smartphone is not the only thing that needs recharging.

The brain does, too!

Source:
Psychology Today: Breaks Help Memory: https://tinyurl.com/yb3y95nd
Go to "Social Triggers:" See under "Why you need to take more breaks."

Immune system

The idea that there's nothing you can do about your immune system is wrong. Fortunately! And the link between the immune system and dementia is of great importance for how to deal with the disease . . . actually, for how we handle each one of the two *individually*.

Below, we point out a number of factors that are important for the preservation and strengthening of our immune system. They all have to do with lifestyle. That is something we can influence, and these factors apply to healthy as well as sick people, for young as well as elderly, for people with dementia as well as those who are not affected by it.

What is the immune system?

The immune system is an extremely complex system of biological structures and processes that are found in an organism (the host), such as a human or an animal. The function of the immune system is to protect the host against disease-causing elements, the so-called pathogens. It does this by mobilizing antibodies against foreign elements.

When the immune system is functioning properly and efficiently, the antibodies are able to identify elements that are foreign to the host.

Vaccinations are used to provide our body a defense against bacteria and viruses. There are many diseases (childhood diseases) we get only once in our life, because the body remembers and recognizes the pathogens from the first time we became ill. It is this recognition that enables the immune system to protect us.

What strengthens the immune system?

Although there are many things we don't know about the immune system, we do know a lot about the factors that can strengthen and weaken it, and that we can control ourselves—typically without thinking about them.

In addition to avoiding the harmful things mentioned below, the three most important positive factors are:

1. Vitamins - Vitamin D is known to be good for strong bones, but it also has a positive effect on the immune system. Fatty fish, eggs, milk and sunlight are our main sources of vitamin D. Vitamins A, C, and E are also important for the immune system. They are found in healthy diets (most plant-based foods), such as fresh vegetables, seeds, and nuts; these are also important for fiber intake. Do not forget ginger and turmeric (as a spice or tea). See the articles on healthy eating in Section 3, p. 47.

2. Exercise and outdoor life - Aerobic exercise helps the body fight diseases, an effect that is associated with good blood circulation. And outdoor life is an added plus. In addition to sunlight, many of the "substances" we breathe - for example in the forests - are also important for the immune system. See the articles about this in Section 3, p. 47.

3. Do not forget sex - It has been documented that bactericidal immunoglobulins (IgA) promote the immune system and that sex is an activity that is important for the formation of IgA - see the fifth article on sex and intimacy (Section 6, p. 139). Weekly intimacy is markedly better than sex more rarely. So, unless sex for other reasons is *not* part of your lifestyle, take advantage of it.

What harms the immune system?

There are also many things to watch out for in order to break down your immune system. Here are the most important:

4. Sleep - We often get sick when we have a permanent lack of sleep (see the article, *Sleep*, p. 78). If we get less than 7-8 hours of sleep - regularly! - the body can not produce enough of the proteins (cytokines) that help the immune system with producing antibodies. Lack of sleep is not just a matter of being tired.

The worst thing is that too little sleep increases the risk that the immune system will not be able to handle the infections we are exposed to. It is therefore one of the first areas you need to pay attention to if your health is deteriorating and there is no obvious explanation for why.

5. Tobacco and alcohol - Nicotine from tobacco products (of any kind) can weaken the immune system. Even vaping and marijuana are harmful in this and other contexts. In addition to nicotine, there are other immune-damaging substances in tobacco products that are inhaled.

One drink too many every day can ruin the body's ability to fight diseases. Maximum daily alcohol intake is one shot for women and two for men. Long time consumption of larger amounts of alcohol can permanently damage the immune system.

6. Poor diet - A diet rich in saturated fatty acids can prevent the white blood cells in their bactericidal function. Over extended periods, a fatty diet can disrupt the microflora of the intestinal system, which can also lead to a weakening of the immune system.

The answer is a diet low in fat and sugar. You get the good fatty acids if you follow the *Mediterranean diet plan*, see p. 54.

Other important factors

The list above is not complete. There are a few other areas we rarely think about in terms of their negative impact on our health. It is therefore important that you are aware of them. They are:

7. Medicines - There may be negative consequences of taking certain medications. Therefore, it is important to talk to your doctor before starting any new medication or making any changes to your current medication - especially if you are treating chronic conditions. Certain medications may counter-act one another, so watch out for that.

8. Stress - It's difficult to do cope about anxiety, nervousness, stress, and grief as they are externally induced threats to our health. These factors are known to have a significant negative impact on the immune system, in fact so dramatic that 30 minutes of severe nervousness can instantly impact our immune system adversely. Add to this mixture the negative impact of stress on your sleep, etc. A vicious circle!

To cope with that, listen to music; read a book; find activities that, by their nature, are soothing; consider meditation - it's something everyone can do.

If you are struggling with anxiety, stress, and grief for extended periods of time, talk to your doctor about it. Each one of them can seriously damage your health.

Inflammations

Changes in life style can either contribute to or hinder a healthier and longer life, but it's not until recently that geriatric research has shown that chronic inflammation is a factor that can harm brain health.

Chronic inflammation (see definition and characteristics below) is an irritation that can appear in virtually all of our organs. It is not uncommon to get such irritations as we get older, but they are not the result of infections.

Rather, they are the result of an inability of the body to remove cells that no longer divide (and thereby renew). These cells are called 'senescent cells.' They are normal cells except they don't divide.

Since they are not removed, they accumulate and start to secrete cytokines, which can lead to inflammation.

But there is good news, too

It has been shown that a number of changes in our lifestyle can reduce and even completely counteract the development of inflammation. It is not surprising for those who follow news about healthy living (Section 3, p. 47) that sleep, diet, exercise, etc. are the most important factors, just as stress reduction, smoking, and an appropriate weight are important, too.

Since stress is less tangible than the other factors, here are a few words about this insidious and all too common condition.

Beware of stress

As mentioned, stress contributes to inflammation. Stress also causes sleep disorders, which in turn can lead to inflammation in a vicious circle that eventually can become chronic.

Often, we cannot change much about stressful situations in life, but we can learn to handle them better by, for example, meditating.

Meditation and yoga are among the lifestyle factors that best counteract stress in everyday life. And mind you, we are *never* too old to start meditation.

Be careful with medication

Finally, it should be mentioned that we need to use medication with caution (see articles on p. 105 and p. 109). There is a tendency to over-medicate ourselves, especially with painkillers. The so-called "non-steroidal anti-inflammatory drugs (NAIDS) can disrupt and destroy the ecology of the microorganisms in the gut and cause bacteria to enter the bloodstream. This can lead to a serious inflammatory condition.

Explanatory note on inflammation (lat.: "ignite a fire") Inflammation refers to the immunological processes the body uses to heal itself when it is exposed to infections, injuries, or toxins and has challenged/damaged our cells.

These processes are often very short-lived (from a few hours to a few days). We therefore call them acute inflammations. The symptoms are usually local pain and swelling with redness.

Chronic inflammation occurs when the response to the challenges lasts for a long time (months and years) but at a lower level. It puts the body on constant alert and can eventually result in damage to tissues and organs.

The symptoms are typically mild and can be easily overlooked. They typically include fatigue, low fever, sore joints, sores or rashes.

For older people with a weakened immune system, chronic inflammation can be extremely harmful.

Sources: National Geographic - Jan. 2020, p.85; and NIH: rapport

L-Serine

What is L-Serine?
L-Serine is a non-essential amino acid that is part of most proteins in our body. It is called non-essential because a healthy body produces enough L-Serine to eliminate the need for it to be supplemented.

Under certain circumstances, the body does not have enough L-Serine. It can happen if we ingest a toxin called BMAA (beta-methyl-amino-alanine), which is formed by cyanobacteria (blue-green algae).

Since we typically do not get in contact with blue-green algae, you may wonder how we possibly might ingesting them. The answer is water pollution.

Most of what we know about BMAA comes from studies done by a man with an unusual background. Dr. Paul Cox is a botanist and not a medical doctor or neurologist. He therefore does not enjoy the professional respect that other doctors/neurologists would have, and many reject his claims on that basis alone.

But Dr. Cox has long been on the trail of this toxin and its possible impact on the development of dementia, ALS (Lou Gehrig's Disease), Parkinson's, autism, and other neurological diseases.

It has therefore become the subject of extensive research.

What do we know?
The L-Serine/BMAA relationship is a very complicated "multi-factor" problem, so we do not know a lot about it yet. But a few things are clear:
- BMAA is a cell toxin
- we have a certain risk that the body absorbs BMAA if the water or the food we eat have been contaminated with blue-green algae

- BMAA prevents L-Serine from being involved in the formation of the fat that surrounds the nerve connections between the neurons in the brain (that works like the plastic insulation of an electrical wire)
- if the insulating fat deteriorates, is in deficit, or is missing completely, the connection between the neurons does not work as well

Experiments with daily intake of 30g/day L-Serine seems to help with brain functions. This is where optimism comes in:

If we can boost the content of L-Serine by a daily intake, we may be able to not only prevent the effect of BMAA but also achieve a protection against neurological diseases such as dementia.

What can we do?

We get L-Serine by eating dairy products, sesame, sunflower , and pumpkin seeds, soy products and other beans, as well as peanuts and pistachio nuts.

We typically do not eat all these products - or not enough - so instead, you can take L-Serine in the form of an amino acid powder (available over the counter). There are no known side effects with L-Serine, but it is always a good idea to consult your doctor before starting to "experiment" with dietary supplements - and tell your doctor why you think it might be helpful for you.

###

PS: For the sake of good order, we should mention that the authors have no commercial interest in L-Serine products.

###

Sources:

NCBI article on L-Serine (https://www.ncbi.nlm.nih.gov/pmc/articles/PMC5615428/

University of Melbourne article on rebuilding myelin in the brain: https://tinyurl.com/y6hba7c9.

Medical drugs - be careful

Frequent use of medical drugs can lead to dementia.
This is why older people need to be vigilant and should talk with their doctors about both their medication - and dementia.

What's the issue?

The use of drugs is a complicated issue and involves a well-known, classic conflict. A drug is good for something but less good (or even harmful) for something else.

In this article we take a look at the substance *acetylcholine*, a biologically active substance that controls a number of bodily (mis)functions like COPD, seasonal allergies, depression, incontinence, and overactive bladder. To alleviate/eliminate problems (avoid "overreaction" in the body) of this kind, doctors often prescribe anticholinergic medication.

That's the good thing.

The bad thing is that acetylcholine also plays a major role in maintaining normal cognitive functions of the brain; therefore, *anticholinergic drugs* may increase the risk of accelerating the decline in cognitive functions in older people. This effect has been documented in countless experiments.

Previous trials and results

A number of trials over the years have established two functions of anticholinergic drugs:

(1) an impairment of the function of the anterior part of the brain, which is where acetylcholine is *produced*, while

(2) a reduction in the body's *"stock"* of acetylcholine

The combination of these two functions is a weakening of our memory and other cognitive functions. As in many other situations, this risk is particularly clear in people with biomarkers for Alzheimer's or other genetic factors that may lead to dementia.

New studies

Recent trials included 688 people over 74 years of age who at the start of the trial had no signs of dementia. One-third of them took at least one type of anticholinergic drugs (with an average of 4.7 drugs per person!) These people were followed for a period of over 10 years and were given annual cognitive tests.

Compared with people who took no anticholinergic drugs, **people who took at least one drug had a 47% increase in the risk of developing a mild degree of dementia.** That risk more than doubled if the person *also* has a genetic disposition for dementia, and the risk was five times higher if the person has biomarkers in the cerebrospinal fluid!

What now?

Experiments also show that by *reducing* the use of anticholinergic drugs, one can defer (or possibly prevent) cognitive impairment.

Considering the widespread usage of such drugs, this is significant. But as pointed out, you take that kind of medicine for a good reason. It is therefore very important to discuss these aspects with your doctor—especially the question of whether you are taking the right dose of anticholinergic (or other) medication. It is not uncommon to be able to cope with other ailments with a smaller dose of medication.

See also the article on *Medicine - do they work?* on p. 109.

Sources:
Research with anticholinergic medicine: adn.loni.usc.edu
MNT, Risk of dementia: https://tinyurl.com/yxgzvv8w
Article in Neurology: https://tinyurl.com/y359q9e6

New medicine for Alzheimer's

There are indications that the long-cherished dream of a drug for Alzheimer's may come true.

The American biotech company, Biogen, has applied for approval to make a new product (aducanumab) ready for marketing in the US and Europe. The application may take 1-2 years, but it is the first promising step on a long road towards a medicine for dementia. As there are no other products on the market that can alleviate Alzheimer's, there are high expectations for this new drug.

The announcement from Biogen was a surprise because the company last year completely stopped working with aducanumab due to disappointing results. But new and much more data from the very same studies show a significant positive effect for people with Alzheimer's.

The effect - and the mechanism

The effect is first and foremost a slowdown in the development of the disease to such an extent that affected people can continue their daily chores and retain their memory for much longer than usual. Aducanumab works by removing the so-called ß-amyloid, a protein which is deposited between the brain cells and which is considered to be toxic to the brain (see the articles in Section 5, p. 121).

There are, of course, other mechanisms involved in the development of dementia, but the removal of amyloid is one of the important ones.

What can we expect?

Any improvement in the condition of people with Alzheimer's is important, and we should welcome all good news. And there has been no good news for over ten years.

But improvements and treatment are not the same as a cure, and in medical research we must not become overly optimistic.

Nevertheless, Biogen hopes that the new product will start a development within the global dementia research community towards more new products, so that within a relatively short time horizon we can have an effective treatment of this serious disease complex.

Aducanumab, is under FDA review for potential approval at this writing.

The very latest (March 2021):
Another product currently is under development, donanemab from Eli Lilly, seems to have a very promising effect in binding the plaque in the brain. Whether this may result in *removing* the plaque from the brain or simply *delaying* any further development of Alzheimer's remains to be seen, but this has made scientists very excited and optimistic.

We will follow this development and bring updates in later version of this book.

Sources:
Biogen press release: https://tinyurl.com/y4pk3zao
and
BBC Health News - https://www.bbc.com/news/health-50137041

Medicine for dementia - do they work?

Although there is currently no cure for dementia, there are medications that can reduce and relieve the symptoms. Using them is one of the ways towards increased independence and zest for life in people living with dementia.

Dementia and medication

The big question is how to preserve the quality of life of people with dementia and ensure they have the best possible quality of life. Without a definite cure, the goal is therefore to reduce the complications of living with dementia and cope with the practical tasks of daily life, incl. strengthening memory, language, etc..

That is in addition to the medication many elderly people take for high blood pressure, depression, and behavioral changes - all to increase their quality of life.

What is available?

The U.S. Food and Drug Administration (FDA) has approved five drugs for the treatment of Alzheimer's:

rivastigmine
galantamine
donepezil
memantine, and
memantine combined with donepezil.

The five ones mentioned are used for various dementia diseases, and it varies *when* in the dementia process it is most appropriate to use them. In general, dementia medicine works for a limited period of time, often only 1-3 years.

However, since all these aspects depend on individual circumstances, discuss with your doctor which medication is best for you.

Remember the medicine!

It may seem superfluous to mention that once the prescription is written, the next step is to take the medication; but taking medicine can be a challenge for people with memory loss.

This is where you can take advantage of memory devices like dosing boxes or medicine dispensers with alarms, which can ensure that the correct dosage of medicine is taken at the right times of the day.

A good piece of advice is to introduce memory systems as early as possible (see p. 36-38). It makes it easier to introduce and maintain the new habit. The earlier a new routine is introduced, the longer it will last.

Professionals know best

Medication is only part of the treatment for people with dementia. It is equally important to provide care and attention as well as exercise and diet. Together, this can help ameliorate the symptoms of dementia and create a better quality of life for a person.

You should always ask a professional for advice if you have questions about medicine and other treatments for a dementia disease.

In the article *Independence* in Section 2, p. 43, you can read more about how to maintain your lifestyle while coping with dementia.

Read also the article: *Medical drugs - be careful!* p. 105.

Menopause

The answer to why three out of four people with Alzheimer's are women is complicated. In this article, we look at what *we think* we know about the differences between men and women . . . and about why there's a link between menopause and dementia.

Small differences - big effects

It is not exactly breaking news that men and women are different; some will say vastly different, others will say less so. But in one area, women are completely different from men: their mid-aged menopause.

We usually focus on finding the cause in the body. We know it's something with the ovaries and decreased hormone production; in other words, changes in the female *body*. And with that focus, we completely overlook that the cause is found in the brain!

That's news to most. Men's and women's brains are generally considered to be exactly the same (at least among brain researchers), but new research shows they are very different in terms of *how* they change during their mid-life years.

Dementia and the brain - a new angle

In short, because men and women have different reproductive systems, we age differently from around 50 years of age. In relation to dementia, it is all about the brain - more precisely the brain's communication with the body. In the period from mid-twenties to menopause, men and women experience roughly the same slow, gradual decline in hormone production. For men, it is primarily testosterone (although men also have estrogens), and for women, it is primarily estrogen (although women also have testosterone).

But from the time around and after menopause, women's estrogen production - especially estradiol - drops dramatically, while men's hormone production continues the gradual decline until well into the 70s. Estradiol plays a major role in supplying the brain cells with glucose (i.e. energy). The decrease in estradiol therefore leads to much lower energy (more than 30%), which, in relation to the brain, means faster aging.

Brain-body dialogue

The latest research shows that the problems related to menopause are functions of lower energy in three areas of the brain:
- *hypothalamus* - which regulates body temperature; with a lower estradiol production (lower energy) women experience hot flashes
- *brainstem* - which plays a role in sleep; with a lower estradiol production (lower energy) women experience difficulty sleeping
- *amygdala* - which plays a role in our mental state; with a lower estradiol production (lower energy) women experience mood swings

And at the same time, these changes lead to the formation of non-soluble amyloid plaque in the brain - a relatively new field of research. It also appears that women's brain cells have a structure that allows a faster spread of the dementia-inducing beta-amyloid.

All together, when women feel 'out of balance,' it is because they are experiencing a new state in the brain's energy function. To emphasize that point, (female) neurologists have therefore shown that ". . . **compared to men, women do not have lower *cognitive* functions *after* menopause - just like they don't have lower cognitive functions *before* menopause** "(Lisa Mosconi).*

Yes, women may be tired, but they are just as sharp as before these changes started.

A completely different aspect

As mentioned, three out of four people with Alzheimer's are women. Besides the biological reason described above, there are a

couple of *sociological* reasons that add to the explanation (Nat. Geo):
- there are fewer women than men in the labor market (people who work are less likely to get dementia because of, among many things, the social interaction with others)
- since most memory tests are word-based tests and women typically are better at remembering words than men are, women go undiagnosed for longer time and the disease is more advanced when they finally *are* diagnosed with dementia

These fields are subject of intense research.

What can you do?

Women can, of course, not do anything about the fact that they all undergo menopausal changes (if they still have their ovaries). Hormone therapy (estrogen) is good for many but often comes with side effects - and there is no evidence that high levels of estradiol prevent Alzheimer's.

But there is good news anyway:

Most physicians will point to the lifestyle changes described in Section 3, p. 47, i.e. diet, exercise, stress and sleep . . . *And do not forget dark chocolate!*

* Don't miss the excellent TEDTalk on menopause by Lisa Mosconi (13 min; English) - link: https://tinyurl.com/y59v76kq

Dizziness

We all experience dizziness from time to time, but we usually don't think much about it. But new research suggests that this is something we need to pay attention and be wary of.

Dizziness, in general

Dizziness is many things, or rather, can have many causes.

All people experience dizziness. This often happens when you get up too quickly from picking something up from the floor or having laced up your shoes. That kind of dizziness is caused by the blood not being able to keep up with the rapid, upwards motion. The brain therefore receives less oxygen - and you become dizzy and lightheaded for less than a minute. With a few deep breaths, it usually passes quickly.

The dizziness we are talking about in this article is associated with a sudden drop in blood pressure while being in an 'upright' position (sitting, standing, walking).

What do we know, what don't we know?

Briefly, researchers conclude that dizziness as early as the age of 50 indicates that people have a higher risk of getting dementia later in life - some mention a 40% higher risk.

But, as said before, this is not the same as saying that dizziness *causes* (will cause) dementia! What we are talking about when we say 'higher risk' is that people with dementia often had dizziness when they were younger.

Researchers admit the reason for this connection is speculative. However, they often talk of an "accumulative effect" - i.e. that the risk increases with an increasing number of "dizziness events." Knowing that dementia cannot (yet) be cured, it is important to find these connections at a time when something possibly can be done about it.

What can and should be done?

If you often experience dizziness, the first step is to talk to your doctor if "something is wrong." Your doctor will not/rarely be able to diagnose dementia at an early stage, but he will look for possible, specific causes for dizziness that should be discussed and treated.

Regulating blood pressure should be something you discuss with your doctor - even if he/she does not raise the issue on his own! The American Academy of Neurology explicitly recommends to measure your blood pressure when you switch from a sitting to a standing position.

Controlling blood pressure can be a way to help preventing or delaying the onset of dementia later in life. If your doctor does not find anything specific during a routine exam, it's up to you to do as much as possible to prevent or postpone the risk of developing dementia later in life through changes in your lifestyle.

It may sound a little overwhelming, but your doctor can point to general things - and you can find a lot of information about this in Section 3, p. 47.

Note:

Our blood pressure is usually indicated by two numbers, eg 120 over 80 mm Hg. The high number is the systolic blood pressure when the heart is pumping, and the low number is the diastolic blood pressure between two heartbeats - see also p. 91.

Researchers talk about low blood pressure if it is lower than 90 over 60 (mm Hg).

Test or not

What are the pros and cons of being tested for Alzheimer's, i.e. the pro and cons of knowing if you're at risk of developing Alzheimer's?

Read about it here - but keep in mind that only you and your relatives can decide if a test is a good idea - for you.

It is not a very long time ago that one could only determine if a patient had Alzheimer's by performing an autopsy. And for those affected, that's a little late! But that has changed!

Now there are brain scans and "spinal taps" (see note 1 below) on the way. These tests can detect the presence of beta-amyloids - the tell-tale sign about Alzheimer's - in the brain. Researchers are also working on a blood test for another protein, the so-called tau protein, which is also characteristic of Alzheimer's. These tests are not available outside the research laboratories yet, but they are close.

That's both exciting and promising . . . or is it?

Difficult questions

As these tests become more common, an important question arises for those who fear their cognitive functions are disappearing: 'Am I sure I'd like to know if Alzheimer's is under development?'

It's a lot easier to want an answer to the question about the gender of the child you expect, so you can choose the name of the child or how to decorate it's room, etc. And if you just knew the Alzheimer's test would be negative, then it's not difficult either.

But, of course, you cannot be sure of that.

For many, balancing the arguments below can be overwhelming, and many aspects come into play in the decision to be tested and get an answer.

I want to know because . . .
- a "positive" test can help me plan for the future and organize and bring 'order' in financial and private matters, such as a will/testament/inheritance
- if I get another serious disease, I can make the decision to let it run its course without treatment
- I can have time to say goodbye to people I perhaps don't see often
- I can get involved in Alzheimer's associations/support groups
- I can try to avoid letting "the disease define who I am" and become an inspiration to others

I don't want to know because . . .
- I can not face the fact that one day I will not be able to recognize my spouse/partner and my children
- I can not face the fact that one day I can not speak
- it's a horrible way to die; I'd rather not know about it for sure
- will and can my spouse/partner support me all the way?
- will friends remain friends?
- now I'll know something I can not "un-know" (forget) again - and it will affect me for the rest of my life

What do the professionals say?

Doctors and psychologists recommend starting a conversation with your spouse/partner and perhaps your children and seeing how you yourself react by simply talking about it - and, of course, seeing how the family responds.

An Alzheimer's researcher at the University of Pennsylvania assuaged his patients by emphasizing that "none of my patients have committed suicide"—meaning that it may be bad, but you can manage it! Along those lines, many people said, in fact, they could now take active steps to delay the development of Alzheimer's (changes in diet, exercise, and sleep, etc.).

But the problem for doctors is often that they don't know themselves what to say to patients. It is not possible to determine for sure whether a patient's impaired memory function is a normal part of getting older, or whether dementia is on its way.

And even with a test that determines amyloid plaque between the brain cells - the typical pathway to Alzheimer's - it can take many years before the disease manifests itself.

Doctors may even suggest postponing a test and saying, "You are OK. You're 75, maybe a little depressed. Let's try something against that. "

So . . . what is best?

That depends entirely on you. No answer is universally good for everyone. It really boils down to the fact that no one outside the circle of your closest family members can give an advice that suits you.

But the sooner you start the conversation, the better!

Notes:

1: "Spinal tap" is a sample of the fluid that flows through the brain and spinal cord. It is used to tell if there is an infection or bleeding in the brain. The sample is taken between the 3rd and 4th lumbar vertebra - and not in the brain.

2: A recent announcement from the biotech company, Biogen, shows that they are well on their way to the first treatment, which can delay the disease if the treatment starts early enough - see the article *New medicine for Alzheimer's*, p. 107.

Source: https://tinyurl.com/y2q4sbkd

Vaccination

As you know, there is no cure for Alzheimer's, and we are not talking about vaccination against Alzheimer's in this article.

Rather, the new, hot subject in science is that vaccinations against pneumonia and influenza have an unexpectedly big advantage: They seem to lower the risk of getting Alzheimer's.

Getting vaccinated against pneumonia and influenza entails all the benefits we are familiar with. But now it has been established that these vaccinations also protect against the development of Alzheimer's.

Studies show a positive correlation. . .

The results of two new (unpublished as per Nov. 2020) studies involving 9,000 and 15,000 people over the age of 60 were presented at the Alzheimer's Association in the United States in early 2020.

In the first group, it was found that those who had received at least one flu vaccination had a 17% lower risk of getting Alzheimer's. Those who received annual vaccinations had an even greater reduction in risk.

In the second group, it was found that people who were vaccinated annually against pneumonia and influenza in the ten-year period between 65 and 75 years had up to 30% lower risk of Alzheimer's.

However, these lower risks were more modest if people had a genetic predisposition to Alzheimer's.

Researchers warn against over-interpreting these results. As always, we have to remind ourselves that a connection/correlation is not the same as the *cause/reason*!

. . . but what *is* the reason?
Now researchers are wondering . . .

(a) whether vaccination against pneumonia and/or the flu affects the *brain* in such a way that it also *protects* against Alzheimer's, or

(b) whether it might be the classic phenomenon in public health that people who get vaccinated have a different lifestyle (more exercise, better diet, etc.) than those who do not.

It is too early to draw conclusions, say the researchers and mention that with COVID-19 (p. 34), the answers to this are perhaps even more important.

Prevention
A third important aspect is that according to Danish studies at "Rigshospitalet" (the University Hospital, Copenhagen), which included more than 1.5 million people, prevention against pneumonia and influenza is critical for people with dementia, because people with dementia have a 6 times greater risk of dying if they get serious infections - a risk that lasts for more than a decade.

So, even though a cause-and-effect relationship has not yet been established, it is important to follow the recommendations of health authorities and one's own physician regarding vaccinations.

Sources:
HealthDay Report: Prevention - https://tinyurl.com/y6nqctmz
as well
Vaccination - https://tinyurl.com/y43a7owo

SECTION 5: ABOUT OUR BRAIN AND OUR SENSES

CONTENTS

1. Dementia and consciousness   page 122
2. Lewy's Body dementia   page 123
3. Myths about the brain   page 127
4. Senses and body functions   page 130
5. Hearing   page 133
6. Vision and hearing   page 136

Dementia and consciousness

From an academic/scientific perspective this article belongs here in the section on *Brain and Senses*, but we chose to place it in Section 1, p. 14 because it *also* deals with attitudes like how we—given the knowledge presented in the article—should relate to people with dementia.

The article presents a whole new view of how the brain and consciousness play together in all people, with or without dementia, and it explains that a person with advanced dementia/Alzheimer's *has the same consciousness as the person had before he/she got the disease.*

If you have not read *Dementia and Consciousness* article yet, we encourage you to go to Section 1, p. 23) and get an eye-opening look into understanding a person with dementia.

There is a lot of food for thoughts.

###

Read for example: *Ordinary People, Extraordinary Experiences.* which is available at amazon.com/books (https://tinyurl.com/mykrt73c). It deals with "new perspectives on consciousness."

Lewy's Body Dementia

Lewy's Body Dementia is the second-most common form of dementia, but it has only come to the forefront in recent years. Read here how Lewy's Body Dementia is different from Alzheimer's (see also the article *Dementia and Alzheimer's* in Section 1, p. 26).

When one of the world's most beloved comedians, Robin Williams (1951-2014), committed suicide, the autopsy showed he had the Lewy's Body Dementia disease. This kind of dementia therefore came to the public's attention.

Although Lewy's Body Dementia in many respects is similar to Alzheimer's, there's a great deal of ignorance about how LBD differs from Alzheimer's disease.

Let's start at the beginning.

Background

Lewy's Body Dementia (hereinafter LBD) was diagnosed in 1914 by Dr. Frederick Lewy, who found an accumulation of proteins in the brain of people with Parkinson's disease. These protein accumulations were later named Lewy's bodies.

Since neither LBD nor Alzheimer's disease (hereinafter AD) can be cured (and only to a certain extent treated), it is reasonable to ask why we are bringing this article. The answer is simple. It's about being prepared. Both diseases progress slowly and irreversibly and almost always end up requiring extensive care.

Our focus is therefore on what distinguishes the two diseases. We hope the information below can help both the person with the disease, their relatives, and therapists.

Differences and similarities
1. **The development**: As mentioned, both LBD and AD cause a slow deterioration of brain function. This makes it difficult

to determine exactly when the disease starts. There is often some overlap with Parkinson's disease, and neurologists often talk about "Dementia With Lewy Bodies" when cognitive functions deteriorate at least one year *earlier* than motor impairment. If cognitive function deteriorates more than one year *after* motor impairment, it is referred to as "Parkinson's With Dementia."

2. **Frequency**: After AD, LBD is the second-most common form of dementia. Approx. 10-20% of all cases of dementia are LBD; there is about 1 person with LBD for every 4 people with AD. LBD often occurs with Parkinson's. While there are far more women than men getting AD, there is a predominance of men with LBD. Both diseases usually start after the age of 65-70, but can start as early as age 50.

3. **Causes**: LBD is caused by an accumulation of "Lewy bodies," a protein called alpha-synuclein. It prevents the communication between the brain cells. AD is characterized by amyloid plaque between the brain cells and an "entanglement" of tau protein inside the brain cells. It is not yet known what starts the construction of these substances.

4. **Brain functions**: The most characteristic features of brain function in a person with LBD are that memory and recognition fluctuate significantly and frequently - often from one day to the next - and deteriorate over time. People with AD, on the other hand, have a gradual, steady deterioration in brain function.

5. **Physical motorics**: Both diseases manifest themselves in the same way: difficulty walking, poor balance, and general impaired control of motor functions. The difference, however, is that these difficulties appear early on in LBD but only quite late in the development of AD.

6. **Facial expressions**: Most people with LBD rarely show their emotions. Incidentally, this is an overlap with people with Parkinson's disease. People with AD first show a

reduced variation in their facial expressions at a much later stage in the development of the disease.
7. **Visual hallucinations**: Hallucinations are very common in people with LBD and, interestingly enough, typically occur in the early stages of the disease. It is rare for people with AD to have hallucinations. If they do occur, it is usually late in the course of the disease.

Is there a test or some medicine?
Tests: There are no specific blood or urine tests for LDB and AD. Many other tests (metabolic panel, thyroid, vitamin B12, Lyme's and HIV) are used to rule out other possibilities for the impaired functions, but the best way to determine LDB and AD is still MRI and CAT scans of the brain.

Medicine: There is no cure for LBD and AD, but doctors often prescribe medication (cholinesterase inhibitors, antipsychotics and antidepressants, sedatives, and dopamine) all of which reduce symptoms and help with well-being, exercise, and learning. People with LBD and AD should talk to their doctor about these remedies as soon as these diseases are suspected. Any help in that regard increases the quality of life.

Other aspects: LBD and AD are difficult diseases to live with. A person with these diseases has an average life expectancy of 5-8 years, and those years are gradually deteriorating in quality. It takes a lot of energy and attention of relatives and caregivers to deal with such patients. That's why we want to repeat something positive, namely . . .

Lifestyle
It is undisputed that much can be done to alleviate and even delay the gradual break down of the brain caused by these two diseases. Talk to your doctor as soon as you (or your family) have a suspicion about developing dementia. If you have not lived an

optimal, healthy lifestyle for many years, NOW is the right time to start. Your future welfare is largely in your own hands.

Note: In the literature, LBD is often called Dementia with Lewy Bodies (DLB)

Sources:
Alzheimer's og Lewy's:
- Article 1: https://tinyurl.com/y34mv4pf
- Article 2: https://tinyurl.com/y6zvqcbw

Beta-amyloider: https://tinyurl.com/y3qh24f5

Myths about the brain

There are many myths about the brain - far too many. Read about some of the most stubborn ones - and about what we do know about the brain . . . and be surprised.

Studies show that 93% of all adults (34 - 75 years) understand the importance of having a healthy brain, but few are aware of what it takes to maintain a healthy brain. One of the most persistent myths about the brain is that it deteriorates with age and that it cannot be changed.

Recent research show, however, that the brain can change at any age. The past decade has uncovered many exciting things about its structure and function.

Rather than go into this research, we will look at the "easy" side of the topic, Myths and facts.

But first a few surprising facts:
- The brain produces enough electricity to make a 40W bulb light up
- Information travels in the brain with a speed of 300 mph
- The brain works optimally with a variety of things at different ages
- Verbal communication is at its best around 60 years of age - time for the not-so-young-anymore to celebrate
- A weight loss of 3-4 lbs improves cognitive functions by lowering inflammations in the body

Myths and Facts

Myth: We use only 10% of the brain! The facts are that we use a very large part of the brain's many special areas for even small, simple activities.

Myth: Older people will inevitably become forgetful. The facts are: Admittedly, certain things slow down and we eventually tend to forget things, but aspects like assessing human character, social communication, and 'diplomacy' actually improve significantly with age.

Myth: Older people cannot learn new things. Facts are that we can learn new things at any age. Some things may take a little longer as we get older (learning a new language), but our brain is astonishingly "plastic," constantly building new brain cells and new pathways if others do not function optimally.

Myth: One is either a right-brain or left-brain person. Facts are that although language is mostly dealt with in the left hemisphere and spatial orientation mostly in the right hemisphere, the vast majority of activities require a large and *balanced* interaction between both halves.

Myth: Solving one crossword a day keeps the brain going. Facts are: If a crossword is all one uses to stimulate the brain, then it's not the case. We need to stimulate many areas of the brain to keep it fresh (conversations, music, play, sports, learning new things, social activities).

Stimulation of the brain

Let's dwell a little on the last fact, as it is especially relevant if you are nervous about whether you are at risk of dementia.

Increased activity means increased stimulation of the frontal cortex, where judgment and decisions belong, and one of the most important forms of stimulation is social activities. We get such stimulation from many things, like . . .
- spending time with children
- having volunteer work
- having leisure time activities
- having duties
- exercising
- meeting many people
- playing an instrument

- reading or writing on a daily basis
- using your hands (gardening, wood work, etc.).

We can rarely do it all, but the good thing about it is that it's not the *duration* of activities that plays the big role, it's the *variation* — and that applies to all ages.

It should also be mentioned that one of the most overlooked factors for stimulation is having a happy relationship, an optimistic partner, a partner who is most often physically active, eats a healthy diet, uses less harmful substances (incl. alcohol), etc.

And it must be emphasized (again) that 7-8 hours of sleep is often mentioned as one of the most important factors for a healthy brain. And perhaps above all else, the common denominator is that the earlier in life one starts with a stimulating lifestyle, the better for brain health . . . AND:

It's never too late to start!

Source:
Nature: Brain stimulus (https://tinyurl.com/u8tacf6)

Senses and body functions

"Dementia - well, isn't it just something with poor memory?" Many people perceive dementia as a disease that only affects memory. But those who live with dementia close up know that dementia affects numerous other aspects of life.

Although dementia quite often manifests itself as loss or deterioration of memory at the onset of a disease, dementia actually affects the entire brain and, in turn, our senses.

In this article, you can read about how the body's senses are impacted when a dementia disease progresses.

The 7 senses of the body

As children, we learn that we have 5 senses, the sense of hearing, sight, touch, taste, and smell. These senses are located in the cerebral cortex along with other cognitive functions that are directed at our surroundings.

But there are two other senses that are critical to normal/healthy functioning. The *body sense* and the *vestibular sense* (which is also called the balance sense). These two senses inform us where we are in relation to our surroundings - from simple things like assessing how high a chair is and how much force one needs to sit on it, to where we should place ourselves in traffic.

One could say that the last two senses support and are supported by the other five senses. As we move and navigate in our surroundings and different environments, our senses work closely together.

Our sense of sight provides input to our body sense of where the chair is. Our sense of touch provides feedback on how hot or cold it is. But it is the body sense that assesses whether one is freezing or sweating. It is also the sense of touch that, through the feet, assesses what surface we walk on. But it is the sense of balance and the sense of body that assesses how to best place the feet in each step we take in relation to the surroundings.

Sensory confusion

If you are healthy, the collaboration between the senses is something we seldom think about and definitely something we take for granted. But think about these situations:

You have a common cold and cannot hear as well as you usually do. Suddenly there may be words or sounds that are lost, and you may have a hard time keeping up with a conversation.

Or you probably have tried to pick up a carton of milk, thinking it was completely full, but in reality was almost empty. Because your brain sets the muscles in your body to lift something heavy, your arm rises in the air with great speed when you lift the carton.

And if you are severely affected by dizziness - and this is not due to the too many alcoholic beverages you had last night - you may be affected by a virus on the balance nerve (ear).

In each of these situations, the body does not receive the signals from the senses as it normally does, and we therefore experience sensory disturbances.

And that is very much how a person with dementia experiences the world.

What to do? Stimulation!

By stimulating the body in different ways, however, one can help a person who experiences sensory disturbances.

For example, massage stimulates blood circulation. Exercises, where you stomp hard on the floor or knock with light movements on the shoulders and elbows, are other examples of useful stimulations.

There are even a number of aids that effectively can relieve bodily restlessness and disorders. It can be a heavy duvet, a blanket with balls in it, or a tight-fitting vest with weight in it.

Security and reassuring behavior

When you have disturbances of the sense of touch, you are often very stressed. People who have challenges with the sense of touch often find it nice to wear several layers of clothing. Therefore, they also do not like to take it off. In the same way as the heavy duvets, blankets and vests, ample clothing can help to give the person with dementia a feeling of 'security.'

One way to help people who suffer from disturbances of the sense of touch is through loving and calming behaviors. It can be a gentle squeeze of the hand or by stroking them gently on the back. You can put a cloth over the shower head to avoid powerful jets of water. Wellness activities such as scalp massage or lubricating hands and feet with a soothing lotion are other good ways to help.

If the person is affected by an impaired sense of balance, there are a large number of special chairs that can improve the balance. Rocking the person gently in a hammock or moving the person back and forth in a large swing also stimulate the sense of balance.

Get help from a professional

As a relative of a person with dementia, you will most often go to great lengths to alleviate the inconveniences and challenges that become part of living with the disease. The senses are part of an extremely complex, interactive system.

It can be difficult to distinguish between serious, long-term disorders such as dementia or simple things like, for instance, a virus infection. Remember that it requires a professional examination of the sensory apparatus to clarify whether it is one or the other - or something completely different.

Hearing

Recent research suggests that hearing and dementia are connected and in ways we would normally not think about. We should, though. The Lancet Commission reports that hearing is one of the most important factors in reducing the risk of getting dementia.

In this article we look at what it means - and what you can do about it.

It is estimated that three-quarters of all people over the age of 70 have some degree of hearing loss. Like gray hair and wrinkles, hearing loss is considered a natural consequence of getting older.

We are seldom even aware of when our hearing is impaired. It is often said that if you do not hear the doorbell, you do not know if it is because no one is ringing the doorbell, or if it is because you actually cannot *hear* the doorbell.

In other words, it is people in your environment who first become aware of your hearing loss!

What is hearing loss?

Hearing loss is defined as a loss of at least 25 decibels in the audible range of hearing frequencies - a somewhat arbitrary but generally accepted limit (see the notes at the bottom of the article).

Despite modern, advanced technology in hearing aids and the great quality of life benefits by using them, it is surprising that only 14% of the adult population use hearing aids - often out of vanity alone.

Alarming research results

It is, of course, an individual decision not to use hearing aids, but there is every reason to reconsider that decision.

It has been shown that hearing loss is an important factor in the development of dementia and Alzheimer's. This in itself is alarming, but the worst thing is that cognitive impairment occurs with even a very modest hearing loss!

This was discovered 30 years ago with a study of 639 elderly, dementia-free people, who were monitored over a period of 12 years. It was documented that there was a clear, "linear" correlation between hearing loss and the degree of dementia that about 10% of the test persons developed during that period. In 2017, a panel of experts at the medical magazine, The Lancet, concluded that of all the factors that can delay or possibly prevent the development of dementia, hearing loss is the most important (see also p. 48).

This is now supported by two new studies involving 6,400 people over the age of 50. They showed that some degree of impaired cognitive functions occur with hearing loss all as little as a few decibels.

It was a great surprise that impaired cognitive functions could be detected at such a small loss of hearing

What is the explanation?

It is not known with certainty why impaired hearing over a long period of time can impair cognitive capacity. In such cases, there is some evidence that the ear sends vague and incomplete information to the cerebral cortex in the forehead, which is the center of reason, decision-making, and memory. Another explanation may be that hearing loss causes atrophy of the brain tissue if it is not "used" (the "use it or lose it" idea).

This may also be related to the fact that people with hearing loss have fewer (or no) social activities, which in itself is a risk of dementia.

Get a hearing test

Having as good a hearing as possible is perhaps the simplest and most effective way to reduce the risk of or delay the development of dementia. We cannot do much about the fact that we hear less well as we get older, but there is no excuse for not *compensating* for this by

(1) being tested for hearing loss

(2) getting a hearing aid - even if you only have a minimal loss of hearing.

Do it now! Hearing loss starts early and never gets better by itself! Even if you are only 40-50 years old, you should at least have a screening done by your doctor.

It only takes a few minutes.

Note: Hearing is expressed in decibels (dB).

Normal conversation has a decibel level of approx. 60, and your TV (normal volume) has approx. 70 dB.

We can rarely hear anything below 10 dB, and what we usually call "very loud" is approx. 100 dB.

An airplane taking off has approx. 120 dB. . . and a rock concert has approx. 130 dB.

Sources:

The Lancet 2020, Vol 396, Issue 10248, p. 413ff - https://tinyurl.com/y6r25eqw and click on Hearing.

JAMA tests: https://tinyurl.com/y6y9noav

The Lancet article: https://tinyurl.com/y8t8mvys

New tests, see NCBI: https://tinyurl.com/y5bksq77

Vision *and* hearing

"**Dobbelt *sensory loss*" (herefter called DSL)—the simultaneous reduction in vision and hearing—increases the risk of dementia considerably.**
The good news is that it's something you can rectify.

1. Reduced vision and hearing increases the risk of dementia

Studies over many years have established that impaired visual and hearing are individual risk factors for the development of dementia, but it is only recently that researchers have shown how much *greater* this risk is if a person has impairment of both senses *at the same time*!

The assessment of vision and hearing in older people can be an indicator of the development of dementia and Alzheimer's; therefore, the treatment of these sensory impairments is of great importance to the individual - and to society.

2. Vision and hearing get worse with age

The fact that hearing and vision gradually deteriorate with age has prompted researchers to investigate whether they are the result of some of the *same* processes that cause the development of dementia.

Such relationships have been unclear in previous study readers.

3. Studies on vision, hearing, and dementia

The latest studies involved more than 2,000 people over the age of 75. None of the people had, or had only to a limited extent, signs of dementia.

At the *start* of the trial, which lasted 8 years . . .
- 72% of them had no signs of vision or hearing loss;
- 15% had reduced vision; and
- 8% had reduced hearing.

- Only 5% had DSL. Of these approx. 100 people, the vast majority were men, and they were often smokers and drank alcohol.

4. Results: Twice the risk of getting dementia

The risk of getting dementia in the 8-years period was
- 14% for the individuals who had no vision and hearing losses
- 17% for the individuals who had either vision loss or hearing loss
- 29% for the individuals who had DSL at the onset

Compared with individuals without visual and hearing impairment, individuals with DSL had approx. twice the risk (100% increased risk) of developing dementia. The trial also showed that individuals with DSL had a 112% increased risk of developing Alzheimer's.

It is interesting to note that the risk could only to a limited extent be related to the *degree* of visual or hearing impairment.

5. Importance of rectifying vision and hearing loss

More research is needed to determine more precisely the role of visual and hearing impairment in the development of dementia, but the experiment shows that different treatments of visual and hearing impairment in the older part of the population — for example, surgeries, aids/prostheses such as glasses and hearing aids, can have a positive impact on the development of dementia.

In view of the great strain the dementia disease has on the individual and *will* have on society over the next 25-30 years, and with the doubling of the number of older people, it is obvious that much can be gained by addressing these problems as early as possible.

It is largely up to professionals to urge older people address these issues.

It is not often that solutions to serious problems and disorders can be so simple.

Do not postpone an examination and testing of your sight and hearing — and do something about it even if you yourself have minor disabilities.

Sources:
This article is based on information from University of Washington Alzheimer's & Dementia.
See also:https://tinyurl.com/ydbt92tr

SECTION 6: SEX AND INTIMACY

CONTENTS

1. Introduction   page 140
2. Sex - Del I: Changes   page 144
3. Sex - Del II: Challenges   page 148
4. Sex - Del III: Possibilities   page 153
5. Sex or no sex   page 158

Introduction

Sex, the elderly, and dementia are rarely discussed in the same context. The fact that these topics - despite our presumed openness - are still taboos, is a huge problem.

This introduction sets the stage for the following four articles.

Sex, the elderly, and dementia

As mentioned in the introduction, there are over 6.2 million people in the U.S. with a dementia and up to 25 million people who are indirectly affected by it.

Society faces a comprehensive problem in every respect, both from the perspective of the individual and in the larger, societal perspective. And when it comes to sex, the elderly, and dementia, this problem is further magnified.

Myths about sex, the elderly, and dementia

Society has for far too long succumbed to the myth that sex is only for the young and healthy. It may seem natural. After all, this is the group that has to reproduce. But the enjoyment of sex is not linked to reproduction. That means older people can have an active sex life long after the reproductive age.

Studies of these taboos also show that more than half of people between the ages of 50 and 80 are happy with their sex life; in fact, many even say it is better than when they were young. This is especially true for older women, who despite less frequent sex activity are able to enjoy it more than when they were younger and wanted to avoid pregnancy.

Sexuality is an integral part of every person's personality. It is a basic need and an aspect of the very essence of being human; it is inseparable from other aspects of life.

Sex life changes over time

Sex and intimacy are identity-preserving and healthy activities in all relationships. All people experience a gradual decline in sexual activity as they age, so it is important to be prepared for those changes. And that is particularly true if one of the parties is affected by dementia.

It is also important to keep in mind that sexuality is not just a matter of intercourse and that sex is not equally important to all people. Intimate relationships can take many different and, over time, completely new forms. It can include touch, closeness, and activities that are expressions of community and security - forms we previously would not have considered sex.

Therefore, the primary advice is to be open to whatever intimacy means to you, and focus on the things that provide satisfaction in the relationship.

The desire and need for sex has the same broad spectrum of intensity, regardless of which group you belong to (young, old, men, women, social status, or other groupings). It is therefore important to emphasize that people who are affected by dementia are *no different* from other groups of people and do not necessarily lose the desire for sex.

Need for reassessment

So there is a lot we need to reconsider.

Many problems in this whole field are linked to lack of knowledge and understanding of the changes that people with dementia can experience to a greater or lesser degree, and how relatives and caregivers can support the person with dementia.

The better prepared, the easier it is to meet changes and adapt to them.

When it comes to maintaining an intimate relationship after one's partner is afflicted with dementia, there is not just one approach that will work for everyone. Therefore, one should always focus on what is best for the parties in their specific situation.

Many new questions
But nonetheless, many people face new and confusing questions about changes in their sex lives after one party has been diagnosed with dementia.

But keep in mind that these changes have nothing to do with you as a human being! There is not just one 'normal' way of behaving in this very personal subject.

Many people find it difficult to discuss sex and intimacy, and it may be easier for some to talk to a trusted friend or a professional who encounters these issues all the time. Questions can also be raised in a support group where members often have similar experiences as you do.

Contents of the four articles
Three articles explain how dementia can affect the sexual feelings, needs, and behaviors of people with dementia and their partners. Suggestions are given as to how partners can respond to these changes.

A fourth article describes the 10 most important physical and physiological benefits of an active sex life.

It must be emphasized that information and recommendations in these articles are not meant to be a substitute for the professional advice you can and should receive from your doctor, social worker, or professional in the municipality.

The contents of these articles are:

Part I: Changes
Adapting to changes in people with dementia
Less or no sexual interest
Increased sexual interest
Challenging sexual behavior

Part II: Challenges
Changes in inhibitions
Adapting to changes in partners
Ways to deal with frustration
Practical things in nursing home situations

Part III: Possibilities
Consent to sexual relations
If one suspects abuse
Entering into new relationships
Maintaining healthy conditions
Healthy sexuality

Sex or no sex
The 10 most important advantages of an active sex life

Sex - Part I: Changes

Sex and dementia is a complicated cocktail. Not only that, sex and dementia individually can be difficult to discuss; together they are almost impossible - but nonetheless necessary.

Sex in different phases of life can be complicated enough, but when dementia becomes part of the everyday life of a couple (or a single person), you are faced with problems and needs for adjustments you are not prepared for.

Some of these challenges are outlined below. Fortunately, not everyone is struggling with these changes, and often they only appear to a lesser degree. But it is important to know them anyway.

1. Dementia, the brain, and sex organ

The brain is our most important (and largest) sex organ!

This is because, the brain is the 'control center' for all our attitudes and emotions, including sexual feelings and inhibitions. Our genitals do not respond, as most believe, to erotic stimuli *without* direct input (order) from the brain. In other words, your desire starts in the brain.

Because dementia affects the brain, especially the frontal cortex, a person with dementia may experience unexpected and unpredictable changes. Depending on which part of the brain is affected most and what medication they are taking, a person with dementia may experience:

- less or no interest in sex
- increased interest in sex
- changes in the ability to perform sexually
- changes in sexual 'manners' – for example, less understanding/empathy for the need of the partner, or even sexual aggressiveness

- changes in inhibitions – individuals might say or do things they never before would have said or done.

Some couples are able to adapt to these changes relatively easily, while others experience varying degrees of irritation, feelings of loss, anger, embarrassment, nervousness, and frustrations.

2. Less or no sexual interest

Some people with dementia - and even their partners - lose the desire for sex even at a young age and may even in the early stage and become completely withdrawn. Although they can often feel reassurance and enjoyment by caresses, kisses and hugs, they can no longer even show signs of affection. Some people accept that sex ceases as long as intimacy and affection continue in *other* ways.

For example, where partners no longer sleep in the same bed, some people with dementia find pleasure in having something else to cuddle up to, such as a soft stuffed animal or a warm water bottle.

If decreased desire for sexual activity causes problems in the relationship, the couple should seek the advice of their doctor. Remember: it may be a result of another physical illness, hormonal imbalance, or depression.

But the crucial thing is that you allow each other to have the sexuality that you each want - without anyone raising an eyebrow.

○ **Mutual respect**

Many feel guilty if they become less interested in sex than their partner. It is important for the other person to respect their choices, and possibly find new ways to maintain intimacy in the relationship. It is also important to find ways to deal with their own sexual frustrations (see Part II, # 8, below).

There can also be physical and even medical reasons for decreased or lack of interest in sex. If you are not in a good shape, are overweight, or have cardiovascular problems, it can affect sexual desire, but medication (e.g. for blood pressure or depression) can also have a negative effect. These are topics that you should discuss with your doctor before giving in to the idea that "sex is history."

3. Increased sexual interest

Some people with dementia experience increased sexual interest. It is welcomed by some partners, while others are unable to live up to the new need. In the latter case, the situation can become difficult for the person with dementia, and some misinterpret signs of normal affection as an invitation to sexual activity. If the need is overwhelming, instead of pure rejection, it can be valuable to find other activities that the partners can do together and that meet the need of the person with dementia.

Some people with dementia can become aggressive if their sexual needs are not met.

This behavior may stem from the person's emotions and interpretation of the situation. A well-considered and sensitive rejection of sexual needs can overcome the situation without violating his/her dignity and feelings. If this is only a temporary situation, it may be a good idea for the parties to keep some distance until the need diminishes or disappears.

◦ **Handling of problems**

It can be a very difficult topic to discuss. If the parties cannot clarify this alone, they should seek the advice of their doctor or another 'advisor'/counselor. Medical treatment can be considered, but only as a last resort.

If the partner feels that he or she (or others) are in danger, he or she should not hesitate to seek help.

If the person with dementia acts in a way that creates tension with caregivers - for example, in situations with the help of bathing and washing - family members may become ashamed and may consider completely refraining from receiving care assistance from outside. It is important that family members share these concerns with professionals/caregivers, as the family will often be able to point out what the person with dementia may or may not like.

4. Provocative sexual conduct

Many couples' sexual relationships will continue in the normal way, but some may find that a partner with dementia may seem cold and absent when they have sex. Other times, immediately after sexual intercourse, a demented person may even forget that they have already had sex. It even happens that the person no longer recognize his/her partner. These situations can be painful experiences for both parties.

If a person with dementia believes another person is their partner, it is important to try to handle the situation in a way that best preserves the person's dignity.

Try to avoid 'accusations' or being offended but instead talk to the person in a calm and explanatory way. It reduces the risk of people being embarrassed or stressed.

- **If it gets out of control**

In rare cases, some people with dementia go through a phase of sexual aggression and repeatedly demand sex from their partner or other people.

In extreme cases, especially if the person with dementia is physically strong and/or has a background of aggressive behavior, the threat of the use of physical force can be difficult to deal with.

While it is important to remember that such behavior typically is the result of changes in perceptions associated with changes in the frontal cortex - which the person cannot control - it is *also* important that partners and caregivers take care of their own safety.

If the partners in a relationship engage in sexual activities that they would rather avoid, it is important to talk to a doctor or counselor.

The same is true if the partners feel there is a risk of violent behavior or abuse.

You can also contact one of the many organizations that deal with these issues.

Sex - Part II: Challenges

Sex can be a challenge in any case, but when dementia becomes part of the life of a couple (or a single person), you may face challenges you are not prepared for.

In this article, we shed light on the challenges you may face in your sex life when dementia becomes part of daily life.

5. Changes in inhibitions

Dementia can reduce a person's inhibitions. This can lead to them "publishing," what are usually private feelings, thoughts, and attitudes - including things that have to do with sex.

Sometimes a person with dementia can completely lose their inhibitions and invite others to have sex, undress, or touch themselves in public space. They can also use words they have never used before and are completely uncharacteristic of the person.

It is important not to overreact or show signs of shock but to divert the person to other activities. Avoid getting angry or arguing. One must never ridicule a person or let them be ashamed. Lead the person to a private area if their inappropriate behavior takes place in public. Be sensitive and reassuring.

Such situations can be humiliating for friends and family. They can also be confusing, stressful, and frustrating for the individual with dementia - especially if he/she cannot understand their behavior is considered inappropriate.

However, these acts rarely involve sexual arousal. What sometimes appears to be of a sexual nature is often an indication of something completely different (a person who is inappropriately undressed may feel too hot or even have forgotten to dress). So, be circumspect in situations like that.

◦ **Show understanding**

Other actions and attitudes, which appear to be of sexual nature, can be caused by:
- discomfort caused by tight-fitting or itchy clothes, or a feeling of being too hot
- boredom or agitation
- expression of a need for physical contact or affection
- misunderstanding of other people's needs and conduct
- erroneous assumption of a stranger being their partner

Some people want to protect a person with dementia from situations where others might make fun of them or might be shocked by their attitudes. Relatives/partners might, for example, ask others, incl. their grandchildren, not to visit the person with dementia. If you think this is necessary, you should discuss it with another person first and reconsider the decision later, as uncomfortable situations like these often change over time.

6. Adapting to changes in partners

When partners of people with dementia describe feelings about the continuation of their sex life, they mention everything from the joy of still being able to have a sexual relationship to the confusion and insecurity of having intimate contact with a person who at times seems to be a stranger. As dementia progresses, the situation might deteriorate:
- a partner who take care of a person with dementia may feel exhausted by their care giving
- a partner might not have the energy nor the desire to enjoy sex at all; that can be frustrating for *both* parties
- a partner may have difficulties imagining themselves having sex with a person with dementia when at the same time having to help them with intimate physical activities such as bathing or toilet visits. That can make the person with dementia feel a loss of dignity and of feelings for themselves and their partner

- many people find it difficult to enjoy a sexual relationship if only a little of their previous relationship remains. It can feel as if sex no longer has any meaning. If so, it is important to provide the person with dementia with plenty of support, encouragement, and affection in any appropriate way
- some people feel that a partner with dementia may be clumsy or even inconsiderate

In all such situations, the parties should proactively find ways to be intimate - whether it involves sex or not.

◦ **Watch out for stress**

Depending on how dementia affects a relationship, some partners continue to sleep in the same bed. Others choose to sleep in separate beds or in separate rooms. If a partner moves to another room, he or she should be aware that it may be a source of stress and insecurity for the person with dementia. It may help to discuss this with a caregiver, visitor, doctor, or, if you have one, a psychologist.

Mundane, everyday conditions, such as knowledge of when and how often people get up at night, can be remedied with certain technical aids.

7. Ways to handle frustration

Problems can arise when one person expresses a greater (or less, of course) interest in having sex than the other person. If this happens, it helps to remember that this is something most people in long-term relationships experience - even without dementia being involved. In that case, you should look for realistic, practical solutions, or find someone you can talk to about it.

People outside of relationships also have sexual needs, and many can become frustrated when they are not met. This is perfectly normal and no one should be judged negatively because they have these feelings.

If you are responsible for caring for people or for taking care of the household for people who live alone, it can be an advantage to talk to a visitator and see if they can point out problem areas. However, for many reasons, the visitator may find it difficult to talk about inappropriate attitudes, but it is important to know their experiences.

◦ **Talk to one another**

There are several ways to reduce accumulated sexual tension - for example, talking about exercise or masturbation can help.

Sometimes sexual the need for closeness, touch, security, acceptance, and warmth, as well as the need to feel special can be confused with a need for sex. Some people find that if these needs are met, their need for sex is reduced.

For example, close, platonic friendships can relieve the need for emotional intimacy; and various forms of therapy such as massage and reflexology involve physical contact, which can be very relaxing.

It should also be mentioned that studies have shown that people who participate in stress reduction based on "mindfulness" and meditation have improved brain activity and are better at dealing with frustrations. This is related to the positive influence on the hippocampus, which is responsible for learning and memory.

8. Practical things in nursing home situations

Living in a sheltered housing, nursing home, or sharing apartment is not a reason for ending your sex life. Talk to a manager or professional about your need to have private time together and how it can be arranged. Ask what training the staff has regarding relationships, sexuality, and sexual health. You may also want answers to questions such as:

- does the nursing home have a "sexuality policy?"
- what happens if an individual shows affection for or sexual interest in another individual at the nursing home - or a staff member?
- are homosexuals treated with the same respect as heterosexuals?
- does the nursing home have a policy on equal rights?

Every nursing home should have an anti-discrimination policy, and you should ask for examples of how it is enforced.

It is important that every resident can express their sexuality in a safe and tolerant environment.

Sex - Part III: Possibilities

Sex and intimacy in different phases of life can be challenging for everyone, but they can also contain new possibilities as one's situation changes. This also applies to indeviduals with dementia.

9. Consent to sexual relations

Every partner - inside or outside a marriage - has the right to *say no* to sexual activities. But when it comes to a partner with dementia, we have not yet fully understood *whether* (and at *what stage* of dementia) one loses the *right to say yes*.

Both parties to a relationship must give consent to have sex. Consent is based on the fact that it is given *without coercion* and that the person is *fully aware* of the decision.

The problem is, of course, that it is not always clear whether a person with dementia is fully aware of giving consent. This is a significant issue that those involved needs to be very aware of. Usually, the criterion for whether a person is fully aware of his or her consent is that he or she:

- has the mental capacity to understand the information (the "invitation" til sex) *well enough* to make the decision for him/herself
- is conscious about the informationen *long enough* to be able to make the decision
- can *communicate* the decision verbally or by sign, incl. body language like nodding, blinking, or squeezing with a hand.

  ◦ **accept or reject**

In some cases, it may seem as if a person with dementia *passively* accepts an "invitation" to sex by giving minimal feedback. Some partners may feel guilty if it is not clear to them whether the person with dementia wants to have sex. This is a complex ethical and legal issue that needs to be addressed - and which may require professional advice.

If a person with dementia is unable to verbally express his or her wishes, it is important that the partners get to know the non-verbal signs and refrain from any signs of hesitation.

Of course, having dementia does not mean that a person always lacks the ability to make their own decisions or understand the consequences of them. But ability is always linked to a specific situation. A person may, for example, lack the ability to make decisions regarding finances or what medication he or she should take, but may very well be able to make decisions for themselves about taking a bath or cooking.

In sexual situations, the primary, decisive criterion is whether the person with dementia is aware of the *identity* of the person they are with and can clearly say no or express their wishes in another way.

10. If you suspect abuse

If you suspect your partner or another person you know may be being abused emotionally or physically, it is important to bring this to the attention of the authorities/police. Sexual abuse of any kind is a criminal act and the authorities should be involved.

Abuse and aggressive sexual behavior - be it from actual violence to forcing a person to watch pornography - is relatively rare, and it's important to emphasize that it does not occur more frequently in people with dementia than in any other group of people.

- **seek help**

If necessary, talk to a professional about it - but do it (as always when it comes to the sex life of others) in a way that takes into account the privacy and dignity of all parties. There is support available from the Alzheimer's Association.

People you might involve in such cases will assess if the parties in the relationship:

i. are comfortable in their relationship
ii. conduct themselves within the limits of their value norms
iii. are willing and capable to give consent to participate in sexual activities

11. Entering new relationships

People with dementia are still able to enter into new and intimate relationships. Family members, and in particular children of individuals with dementia, can often feel uncomfortable knowing their parents still have sexual needs. But the family must refrain from interfering in this situation if the person really wants to enter into a new relationship that is not to the detriment of any of the parties. As long as the person with dementia has the mental capacity to make such a decision, it is important to respect the person's wishes (see #9, "Consent to Sexual Relationships" above).

- **show respect**

A new relationship is a theme with many variations. There are many positive and life-affirming examples of how people with dementia fall in love and move in together (in care centers) - even if they still have spouses.

The "opposite" is also the case: That a person whose spouse with dementia is still alive, finds a new partner.

These are aspects of infidelity that we are rarely confronted with and dealing with them require great tact and understanding.

For some, it's even a question of whether it's infidelity at all.

It is important that all parties in these matters are treated with dignity and respect, and that the person with dementia does not become the loser because of his or her situation.

It may be a good idea to have an independent advisor to guide the parties through such situations.

- **watch out for difficulties**

But difficulties can arise. For example, it may be that the person with dementia is being exploited by people who have financial motives. It can happen if a former partner (after the end of the relationship) continues to take care of the interests of the person with dementia. It is therefore important that the people involved seek the advice of an independent third party who can facilitate a dialogue about what the parties want.

12. Maintaining healthy relationships

A life with dementia is a challenge, especially at an early stage of the condition. However, there is a lot one can do to maintain a positive relationship.

Separate social activities are useful, but so are activities that both parties can participate in together.

Both promote a sense of self-worth. Participating in activities as a couple or other family unit can also help the person with dementia focus on the positive aspects of the relationship.

It can be as simple things as making a photo album together, listening to music or watching movies together, joining a social group in the neighborhood, finding a hobby you can share, or going on excursions together.

○ **have many conversations**

It is important that both parties have ample support and help in the adjustment phase. If you are concerned or agitated about something, discuss it with:
- people you are close to and who understand the situationen, such as family members and friends
- a doctor, social worker, or home care professional who can often explain the changes the parties face
- a therapist/psychologist (get a referral from your doctor)
- 'helpline' advisors who are trained in giving information and advice and point you toward other organisations where you can get help

And don't forget that if *you* are a private caregiver, it might be a good idea to seeks help and support for *yourself* in a support group or from others who are familiar with situations similar to yours.

13. Health and sexuality

Health problems and medications can have an effect on sexual activity and satisfaction. If one of the parties suffers from painful osteoarthritis, a physiotherapist may suggest ways in which sex can be practiced more comfortably. If one of the parties has had a recent operation or heart problems, one should seek the advice of a doctor before starting to have sex again. The person with such problems may need a waiting period.

Sexually active people are - regardless of age - exposed to sexually transmitted diseases. In fact, the risk is greater for older people. Any signs of unusual itching, discomfort, discharge, blisters, blemishes or nodules around the genitals should be checked by your doctor. One must be aware that many people can have sexually transmitted diseases without having signs of it, and it is therefore recommended to be tested if you have unprotected sex with someone other than one's long-term partner. Good sex hygiene is critical at all ages.

Anyone starting a new sexual relationship should have an open talk about safe sex. Talk to a doctor or seek out information through other health sources as a start to such conversations.

Read also the following article, *Sex or no sex*.

Sex or no sex

Or as Shakespeare would have said: "To have or not to have sex, that is the question."

In this context, that question could be rephrased into 'is it a good idea to have sex when you get older?'

It is rare for a couple (or one party alone) to make the decision to no longer have sex (unless there are specific reasons for it). Rather, what happens is, that sex is "something" which is slowly pushed into the background as you get older.

Before that happens, and before "no more sex" becomes the norm, it is important to know what you're giving up.

Here are the 10 most significant physical/physiological impacts of having sex.

The good news
1. **In general:** People who have sex regularly have a better life . . . physically and mentally.

Researchers in many fields agree that regular sex is important for a healthy body and soul. A strong indication of this is the fact that sexually active people use less medication than those who are less active.

2. Sex is good for the memory

It has been proven that sex promotes memory in people between 50 and 89 years of age. It is not known precisely why, but there are many hints about a connection. One is the connection between sex and the formation of new brain cells.

Also, people over 50 with an active sex life are clearly better able to remember phone numbers, solve math problems, etc.

It applies to both sexes, but is most pronounced among men.

3. Sex strengthens the immune system.

Regular sex raises IgA (immunoglobulin A), which is important in the fight against inflammations and infections. It has been shown that people (young people in this case) who had sex two or more times a week had a significantly higher content of IgA antibodies in their saliva than those who had sex less often.

4. Lower levels of nervousness and stress

Sex reduces adrenaline, the hormone the body produces in stressful situations. Without being able to explain why, researchers have shown that this effect only shows up in sex with a *partner*.

5. Sex is an important factor against depression . . . not just because it is the source of a good relationship, but because sex, and especially orgasm, triggers a high level of endorphins and oxytocin. Women also get an extra high estrogen content, which is good for the health (see also the article on *Menopause* in Section 4, p. 111).

These and other hormones soothe pain (headache/migraine, back, and leg pain) and they help against arthritis and, some say, against menstrual cramps.

There's more good news

6. Less risk of heart diseases. Research shows that people who have sex more often than once a month get heart disease less often than less active people. One of the reasons for that is you get exercise.

And the heart is a muscle that needs exercise. The body burns about 5 calories per minute by having sex. It is almost as much as 100 meters brisk walk. So, half an hour of sex equals 2 miles (3 km) of brisk walking.

At the same time, the body absorbs more oxygen and the blood pressure drops. In other words, if the weather is too bad for a walk, then . . . well, you got the point.

7. Better sleep is an indisputable positive result of having sex (with or without orgasm). Endorphins, oxytocin and prolactin are released and cause one to relax and fall asleep faster. This is especially true for men - something most women can attest to without being scientists!

Sleep (see the article on *Sleep* in Section 3, p. 78) is also critical for mental health, memory, and other brain functions.

8. A longer life is often mentioned as a result of achieving orgasm, especially for women. It is not known why - and one could argue that it is because such people are generally healthier . . . but why take the chance?

9. Prostate health is often mentioned as a result of sexual activity (with orgasm). Although the prostrate gland is involved in the production, and frequent sex therefore could be considered a form of "exercise," researchers are not quite sure why ejaculations have that effect . . . but the cause is not as important as the effect.

10. Sex keep the weight down.

Whether it's because sex makes one thinner or because thinner people have more sex, is not shown. But no matter what, it's a good "side effect."

If sex in itself is not a good enough reason to cultivate it regularly, then all the mentioned benefits are it.

So, to answer Shakespeare's question . . . Yes! It's a very good idea to have sex when you get older - as well as when you are young!

Having said all that, it should, for the sake of good order, be emphasized that sex is many things and not just a matter of intercourse. Closeness, security and comfort, and caresses - something we would often not call sex - are very satisfying for many people.

NOTE 1: All these benefits are of general nature and will not be experienced by everyone. Also, the recommendations here should not be interpreted as medical advice.

Source:
WebMD slides-serie: https://tinyurl.com/yy5jdty4

SECTION 7: ABOUT THE AUTHORS

CONTENTS

1. About the authors   page 164
2. Contact information   page 165

About the authors

Torben Riise, Esther Davidsen, and **Maria Tønnersen** are the main contributors and editors of this book.

Other writers, **Camilla Welling Andersen, Mia Dahl, Christina Jacobsen,** and **Gry Segoli** contributed with several articles and input with professionalism and creativity. For this we are very grateful.

Torben Riise - a native of Denmark with a PhD in biotechnology and an MBA in business economics. He has had a long executive career in international biotech companies in Denmark and the USA. In 1991, Torben started his own international consulting business in Florida. He's currently involved in several social restructuring projects in Denmark.

Torben currently lives in Phoenix, Arizona. He is the author of 7 other books, see https://www.torbenriise.com.

Esther Davidsen - MA (political science), MBA (business), EMCC (certified coach). Esther has had a long career in Brussels, Belgium as an international lobbyist and representative for Region Zealand and the Municipality of Copenhagen. She specializes in health innovation in the EU context, and after moving back to Denmark in 2017, Esther has been involved in several platforms related to 'welfare technoloy' and information technology.

Maria Tønnersen - RN, has a diploma in management and is on her way to earn a masters degree in business and marketing. She has her own company, Demensliv (www.demensliv.dk) in the field of dementia. She is the author of two other Danish books (with co-authors) *Dementia Life - Because life must be lived, also with dementia* as well as *Relatives - Jewels in hiding*.

Contact information

Torben Riise: exec.kaizen@gmail.com
Esther Davidsen: esther.davidsen@hotmail.com
Maria Tønnersen: maria@demensliv.dk

www.ingramcontent.com/pod-product-compliance
Lightning Source LLC
Chambersburg PA
CBHW060838220526
45466CB00003B/1158